DIVERTICULITIS COOKBOOK

300+ HEALTHY LOW-RESIDUE, HIGH-FIBER RECIPES TO IMPROVE YOUR GUT HEALTH AND HEAL YOUR DIGESTIVE SYSTEM. INCLUDING A 100-DAY EATING PLAN TO AVOID THE HASSLE OF SURGERY

Dr. Lindsay Burton

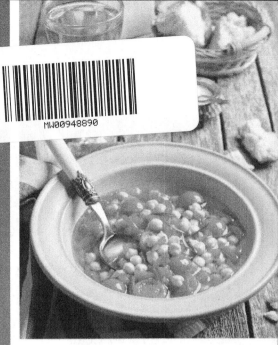

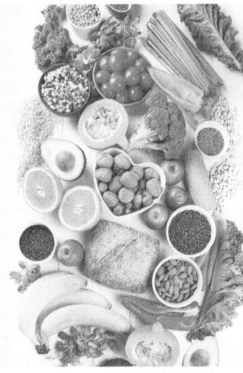

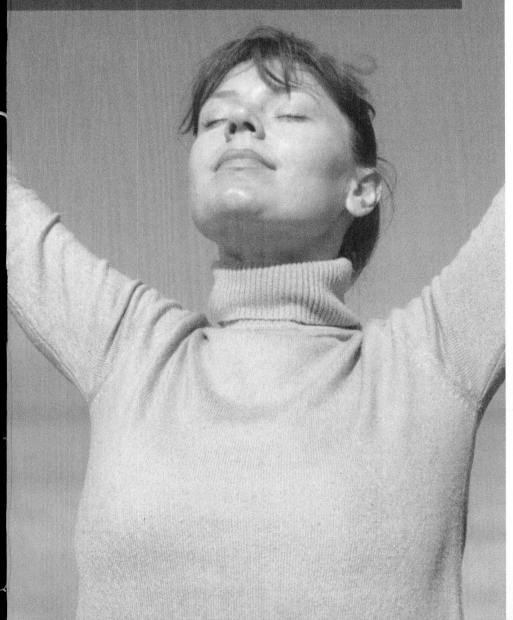

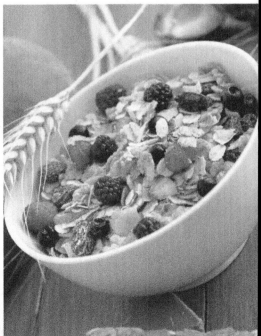

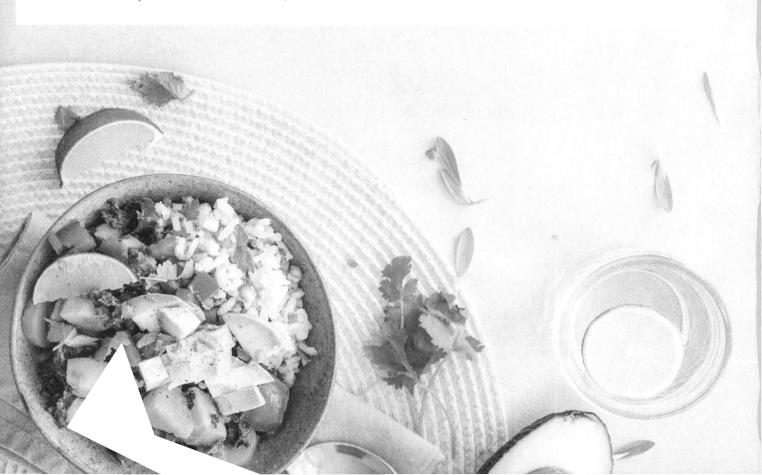

Table of Contents

Introduction

Diverticulitis describes a condition in which pieces of the colon start to bulge out through weakened areas of the intestinal walls. This is a serious illness with an estimated prevalence of 15% among adults in industrialized countries and 6% among young adults aged 20–39. An individual with diverticulitis is much more likely to experience complications, such as bowel obstruction if left untreated, but it can be treated effectively without major surgery.

One way to prevent diverticulitis is by making sure you do not have any heartburn or stomach pain that lasts for more than two hours at a time and does not improve after eating certain foods. If you have diverticulitis, you should drink plenty of fluids and also avoid eating large amounts of fatty foods and spicy foods.

Diverticular Disease Explained

Diverticulosis is a condition that involves the formation of numerous tiny diverticula (pouches or sacs) in the lining of the bowel. These pockets are formed when there's increased pressure on the weak spots of intestinal walls that are caused by waste, gas, or liquid. Diverticular can develop when you are straining when passing stool, especially if you are constipated.

Diverticula mostly form in the lower portion of the colon, known as the sigmoid colon, as a result of it working overtime trying to push out hardened waste or eating very little food. With our diet becoming more and more fiber deficient, diverticula are becoming increasingly common. As per the latest statistics, 10 percent of the people over age 40 and 50 percent of people over age 60 have diverticulosis. But, it's important to note that most people with diverticulosis will have very few or even no symptoms.

Diverticulitis bleeding

This occurs when diverticulitis is not addressed or becomes severely infected to the point that the diverticular walls start bleeding. It is very painful, and the main symptom is traces of blood in the stool.

Can I get Diverticulitis?

Before the twentieth century, diverticular disease was one of the rarest diseases, but today, it has become really common, especially in the Western world.

In the United States alone, it affects approximately half of all people who are above 60 years of age and almost everyone who is 80 years and above. As we get older, the pouches in our digestive tract start becoming more and more prominent.

If you are under 40 years of age, it is very unlikely that you are going to develop diverticulosis unless your diet is very low on fiber or unless you deprive yourself nutritionally by eating way lower than the recommended intake. Diverticulosis also develops in people who do not take a high fiber diet, and that is why it is very common in Western countries as the diet is not rich in fiber and not in Asia or Africa as their diet is high in fiber.

Chapter 1.   What is diverticulitis.

Diverticular Disease, also referred to as, Diverticulitis, is an illness that causes tiny, inflamed sac-like pouches form on your intestinal walls. These sacs protrude through the colon's outer walls creating pockets known as diverticula.

This disease can be considered a silent killer as it entirely possible for it to be present yet undetected if the symptoms are mild. The symptoms could be as mild as light diarrhea or even constipation which can be mistaken as normal. These symptoms would continue to worsen until it develops into your first flare.

As the disease progresses, it goes through various stages. Each stage creating more diverticula (the small pouches mentioned earlier) causing some patients to suffer from thousands of small sacs that grow in size. On the flip side, there are also many patients that only have a single small sac (known as a diverticulum) generally with a diameter of less than a centimeter, though the possibility exists of the sac multiplying or growing over time.

The Latest Science on Diverticulitis

Over the past few years there have been a number of studies into the causes, symptoms, and possible treatments for diverticulitis. In the past five years, more and more countries have issued guidelines on Diverticulitis D with differences regarding covered topics and recommendations including treatments. Presently, there is a lack of certainty on the impact of different drugs on patients who suffer from asymptomatic diverticulosis. A silver lining, however, is that throughout the years of research, limited indications have suggested that a progressive increase in dietary fiber aids in reducing the risk of developing Diverticulitis.

The Diet Stages

There are three main stages to the diverticulitis diet: managing an active flare-up, recovering from it, and preventing it in the future. Throughout each step, you must listen to your body and make diet adjustments slowly, adding one or two new foods at a time while closely monitoring your symptoms.

During a Flare-Up: Clear Fluids

If your flare-up symptoms are extreme, you may need to give your bowel a period of rest. A clear fluid diet will help your body recuperate because it may be temporarily unable to tolerate any solid foods. Take note that this is not meant to be a long-term diet—you should follow it for only a couple of days. Restricting yourself to a clear fluid diet for any length of time may cause you to feel weak, light-headed, exhausted, and hungry. Other symptoms include excessive weight loss, muscle wasting, and depletion of vitamins and minerals. These symptoms occur because it's challenging to meet the body's daily caloric requirements for protein, carbohydrates, and fat through a clear fluid diet. To provide your body with enough energy, you need to consume at least 200 grams of carbohydrates throughout the day. If you have blood sugar challenges such as low blood sugar or diabetes, you may want to monitor your blood sugars during this stage.

After a Flare-Up: Low-Residue Foods

A low-residue (or low-fiber) diet acts as the reintroduction phase, after your flare-up symptoms have mostly passed but before your body is ready for high-fiber foods. "Residue" is the indigestible fiber that passes through the large intestine and then is excreted as a stool. This diet aims to reduce the number of bowel movements you have, which will, in turn, decrease the pain associated with the flare-up. Like the precise fluid stage, the low-residue diet is not meant to be a long-term lifestyle. You should only follow it while you are recovering from inflammation and flare-up pain. Once the pain subsides, you can start introducing more high-fiber foods, working your way up to a high-fiber diet.

Flare-Up Prevention: High-Fiber Foods

This final stage of the diverticulitis diet is the maintenance and prevention phase—in other words, your regular eating routine. When you're not suffering or recovering from a flare-up, a high-fiber diet can protect against the development of diverticula by keeping bowel movements stable and accessible. However, you do not want to go from a low-fiber diet straight to a high-fiber diet, as this can damage your colon. Slow and steady is the rule when it comes to fiber increase: Aim to increase your fiber intake by 2 to 4 grams per week until you reach the recommended amount for your age and biology. Keep in mind that as you increase your fiber.

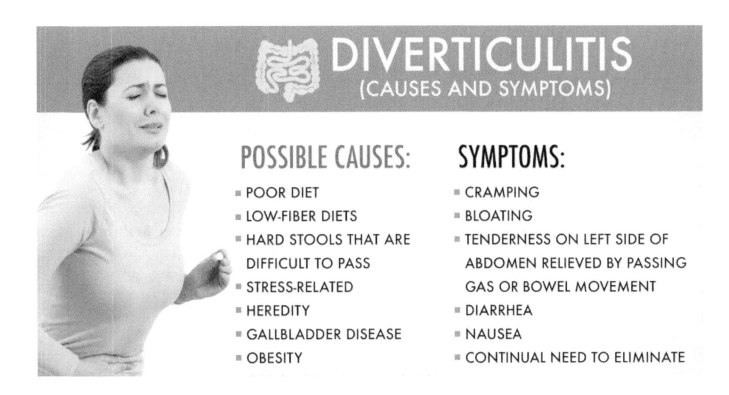

DIVERTICULITIS
(CAUSES AND SYMPTOMS)

POSSIBLE CAUSES:
- POOR DIET
- LOW-FIBER DIETS
- HARD STOOLS THAT ARE DIFFICULT TO PASS
- STRESS-RELATED
- HEREDITY
- GALLBLADDER DISEASE
- OBESITY

SYMPTOMS:
- CRAMPING
- BLOATING
- TENDERNESS ON LEFT SIDE OF ABDOMEN RELIEVED BY PASSING GAS OR BOWEL MOVEMENT
- DIARRHEA
- NAUSEA
- CONTINUAL NEED TO ELIMINATE

Chapter 2.   Symptoms and possible causes.

A majority of the time, diverticulitis is caused by a large amount of waste in the lower part of your bowel due to disease, bacterial infection, physical trauma, or major change in diet. The enlarged pouch becomes inflamed and this can cause inflammation and bleeding into other organs within your abdomen. Diverticulitis can occur anywhere in the large intestine but causes symptoms such as gas pain under the ribs, fever, diarrhea that lasts for more than two weeks without improvement, and abdominal tenderness.

Causes of Diverticulitis

Diet and Intestinal Bacteria

About 90% of people with diverticulitis suffer from chronic constipation. For otherwise healthy patients, it is nearly always caused by a diet low in fiber, which can make the stool too large for the intestine to handle. Also, it's important to know that a large number of people have developed diverticulosis-like symptoms on an all-meat diet. This condition is known as "rabbit starvation" and has been documented throughout history in areas where rabbits are the primary food source.

Past Medical History

People who have had an intestinal perforation or surgery for colorectal cancer are also at a higher risk of developing diverticulosis and diverticulitis.

Age

People under the age of 60 have a higher risk of developing diverticulitis than people over the age of 60.

Hemorrhoids and Clogged Pouches

The development of the condition is in part caused by hemorrhoids, also known as piles, which are enlarged veins in the bottom chamber of your rectum. People with these conditions may have lower levels of internal pressure that can lead to pouching or squeezing off small sacs from within the large intestine. It's also possible for a blockage to form when blood collects inside a small blood vein or artery and leaks into that sac and causes it to swell.

Family History

If your family has been affected by diverticulosis or diverticulitis, you're at a higher risk for developing it than someone who doesn't have this history. It is important to mention that most people with this condition will never develop diverticulitis.

Pregnancy

During pregnancy, a woman's body releases a hormone that causes the colon to relax and allows even small particles to travel more easily through it. This can cause a pouching effect within the large intestine, which can lead to diverticulitis.

Physical Trauma

Fecal matter can become trapped in partial obstruction and this can cause an inflammatory reaction.

Symptoms of Diverticulitis

Abdominal Pain

Diverticulitis pain is often located near the belly button and can sometimes move to either side of the belly. It may resemble a tummy ache, but unlike an upset stomach, it comes and goes.

Fever

You may also experience a fever, which can be mild or high. Your doctor will need to understand if you have ever been diagnosed with diverticulitis, as this condition requires immediate medical attention.

Bleeding

Diverticula can rupture and bleed into neighboring organs like the colon or bladder, or into the abdominal cavity itself. It's not uncommon for some people to pass blood in their stools without knowing that it came from their intestines. Throbbing pain, fever, and nausea can point to an intestinal rupture.

Diarrhea

Diverticulitis can cause diarrhea that is sometimes watery with mucus or blood, according to the National Digestive Diseases Information Clearinghouse (NDDIC). You should see your doctor if you have diarrhea that lasts for more than two weeks without improvement.

Weight Loss

Weight loss and eating a low-fiber diet can lead to diverticulosis and many people may not know until there's a complication like diverticulitis. You need to bring any of these symptoms to your doctor's attention as soon as you notice them because they may be pointing to another serious disease.

Stool Changes

You may notice fluctuations in your stools, such as more than usual mucus, which may indicate a buildup of bacteria or inflammatory material. It is also possible to have a blockage in your intestines that can lead to constipation and cause this extra mucus.

Other symptoms include abdominal swelling that persists after you've passed stool, difficulty breathing or swallowing, the urge to defecate but not being able to do so, and blood in your stool.

How to Know If You Have Diverticulitis

Diverticulitis is a condition of swelling and inflammation of the pouches in the large intestine, which causes pockets to form and can be painful. There are methods for testing to know if you have diverticulitis. Some of these include anorectal manometry, computerized tomography (CT) scan, barium enema, colonoscopy, sigmoidoscopy with biopsy.

If your doctor recommends any of these tests or procedures then you may want to talk about what options you would like and how much they will cost. Let us talk about each of these in detail:

Anorectal Manometry

Anorectal manometry is a test used to measure the function of your muscles around the anus. It measures how well you empty your bowels and if the muscles are working properly. The test involves inserting a thin, flexible tube into your anus and rectum. The tube has no sharp edges or wires, so it shouldn't hurt to insert the tube, but your doctor may give you an anesthetic gel to put on the tip before inserting it.

Computerized Tomography (CT) Scan

A CT scan is a diagnostic imaging procedure that uses X-rays and computer technology to produce highly detailed images of one or more specific areas of an object. You may get a CT scan before or after certain tests such as colonoscopy or sigmoidoscopy. This test is very important because it can detect any abnormalities in the areas that your doctor suspects are infected.

Barium Enema

A barium enema is an X-ray exam of the large intestine and rectum. It's usually performed to see if you have some type of infection or injury in these areas and also to see if there are any problems with your intestines and rectum. Barium is a white, chalky substance that coats the inside of the intestine. When barium is swallowed, it shows up on an X-ray image.

Colonoscopy

A colonoscopy is a procedure used to look at the inside of your colon and rectum through a narrow tube with a camera on the end to see if there are any abnormal growths or infections there. During this procedure, your doctor will insert the tube into your large intestine through your anus and take pictures as they pass along. This test can help doctors determine if you have diverticulitis or another type of infection in the intestines; usually, your doctor won't know for sure until they actually see it during this test. If you're healthy, your doctor may recommend this test if you have high fevers or pain with your movements that lasts for more than 3 days.

This procedure is also done if the doctor suspects polyps (small growths) in your colon or rectum. Polyps are usually harmless but can increase the risk of developing cancer. But, if you have diverticulitis, there's a chance that IBD (Inflammatory Bowel Disease) could develop after the diagnosis of diverticulitis.

Sometimes your doctor may recommend a colonoscopy even if they don't suspect something is wrong because it can help them find out what is making you sick. But, if you already have diverticulitis, then this is not recommended.

Sigmoidoscopy

Sigmoidoscopy with biopsy is the most frequent test that doctors recommend to people who have pain with bowel movements or any other symptoms of diverticulitis. This test involves passing a thin flexible tube into the colon through the anus and turning it so its tip points towards your rectum.

The doctor will look at the walls of your colon with a special instrument called a sigmoidoscope, which can show abnormalities in the lining of your colon. This test can detect signs of diverticulitis, polyps, inflammation, scar tissue, or cancer.

Many people with diverticulitis may be recommended to get this test because it's the most useful to know what is causing the problem if you can have it done by a doctor who has special training in treating IBD.

But if you have diverticulitis then your doctor will just recommend this test without needing to know any other information about you other than that you have diverticulitis. The doctor might also recommend this test if you have had an appendectomy or an abdominal operation in the last 6 months.

Sigmoidoscopy With Biopsy

This is the same test as sigmoidoscopy with a biopsy but it also involves taking small samples of tissue (biopsies) from certain parts of your colon to check for any abnormalities. Colonoscopy is usually recommended first to investigate diverticulitis, but if you have severe symptoms or if you are not able to pass a large amount of stool, then sigmoidoscopy may be recommended before endoscopic examination because this procedure can induce spasms and cause more pain.

Bowel Capsule (H Capsule)

The H-capsule test is done after you take a laxative, and then your doctor will insert an X-ray camera into the anus and rectum to take X-rays of your digestive system while it's working. It's usually performed to see if you have any problems with your large intestine such as ulcers or diverticulitis. This test is more used for gathering information on constipation than diverticulitis. But if you do have diverticulitis, then the doctor might report having extra pressure in the colon or inflammation in the lining of the colon.

Endoscopy

Endoscopy, or gastroscopy, lets the doctor look at the inside of your digestive tract. This test can be done after you have had a biopsy or after you have had an exploratory procedure such as sigmoidoscopy. Endoscopy is usually done in a hospital to allow intravenous sedation and to provide oxygen, fluids, antibiotics, and other medications for the patient. They may also give you medicine to prevent nausea in the operating room. An endoscope is a thin flexible tube with a camera at one end that can be inserted into your rectum or anus.

Chapter 3. How to manage diverticulitis

How to Improve Gut Flora and Heal Your Digestive System

The human body is comprised of over 40 trillion bacteria that have multiple purposes, several of which reside in your intestines. The good bacteria as a collective are referred to as the gut microbiota or gut flora, and they play an extremely vital part in maintaining your overall health. The bad bacteria that form, on the other hand, contribute to many different diseases.

Due to this, you must take care of your gut to ensure that most of the bacteria residing in your body are good bacteria. As you may have already guessed, the food you consume plays a significant role in the type of bacteria that grow inside you.

Maintaining Bacterial Balance

One of the symptoms that are very common in diverticulitis patients is intestinal bacterial overgrowth. That is an overgrowth of harmful bacteria that leads to inflammation and damage to the entire system and makes the entire digestion less effective. Rifaximin is a drug that has been shown to affect this issue positively by returning the bacterial balance to a more normal level. There are also simple foods that will do this as well, including some specialty yogurts. The human digestive field is home to a vast array of bacteria, all of which help digest food. While some bacteria are helpful, many can cause infection and disease, such as food poisoning or diverticulitis. One way to maintain a healthy balance between beneficial and harmful bacteria is by eating probiotic-rich foods. Probiotics are live yeast or bacteria that have been shown to restore a healthy balance of harmful and helpful bacteria in the intestine. Unfortunately, most people do not take probiotic preparations daily. However, studies have shown that taking some form of probiotics regularly can help lower levels of harmful bacteria and restore an average balance between beneficial and harmful bacteria in the gut.

Also, eating foods with higher amounts of probiotics may prevent or reduce the risk of diverticulitis. Brewed foods such as yogurt, kefir, sauerkraut, and kimchi are rich in probiotic bacteria and may improve the balance of harmful to helpful bacteria in the digestive tract. Fermented vegetables such as pickled okra may also help restore an average balance of beneficial and harmful bacteria in the gut.

Take Related Supplements

A person suffering from diverticulitis may be able to find some significant relief by taking probiotic supplements. In combination with other treatments, the probiotic nutrients can give a person a whole new lease on life. Some great food choices already include probiotics in them for example eating foods with kefir, kimchi, or kombucha in them will naturally help reduce the effects of diverticulitis.

Adding a supplement like Prescript-Assist or VSL#3 is not a bad idea no matter where your health is currently at because it will improve your digestion and allow you to feel healthier each day.

Probiotics

It is important to make sure probiotics are in your diet. Probiotics will add healthy bacteria to the digestive system and make the colon work smoother and more efficiently which will allow for less development of diverticular disease. Probiotics enhance the ability of the body to take the nutrients from food, break down lactose, and even help improve the immune system of the body. Low-fat yogurt and kefir are great sources of probiotics for people to consume to avoid diverticular disease.

Prebiotics are another option when it comes to correcting the level of good/bad bacteria in the digestive system. These are substances that are known to develop and nurture the growth and development of the positive forms of bacteria that will keep you healthy and manage your wellbeing.

This is exactly what a person is looking for when they need to restore a healthy bacterial balance. One great probiotic is fructose-oligosaccharide powder but you need to consult a doctor or physician to learn about more prebiotics that can help in solving a poor bacterial balance and help to stop diverticulitis before it begins.

Eat Regularly

It is important to develop a normal eating schedule each day. It is believed that eating all of your snacks and meals at the same time each day will allow for your digestive system and colon to work more regularly and that will keep your colon in great shape and avoid the development of diverticular disease. Make a goal to have your main three meals at about the same time each day along with any snacks. Most people are creatures of habit and this can become easy to do.

Lean Meats

If you are going to consume meats, ensure that they are lean meats. Meats that have an excess of fatty tissue in them are not healthy for digestion and they can introduce too much of the unhealthy kinds of bacteria in the colon, a perceived cause of diverticulitis. Some smart meats to eat are skinless poultry, pork loin, and select lean cuts of steak.

Multivitamins

Post-surgical recovery in diverticulitis is accompanied by the intake of extremely liquid diets that may not completely fulfill the need for vitamin needs of the body. Hence it is very important to make sure that the deficiency is being made through the intake of an additional multivitamin. One should carefully opt for the varieties that comprise naturally grown ingredients that will eventually positively affect our bodies.

The varieties made from food-based supplements are what one should advisably look for. If one takes artificial supplements made of synthetic ingredients, they might just make the medical condition even worse.

Use of Colloidal Silver

When one talks of home and natural remedies for the treatment of diverticulitis, colloidal silver emerges as a promising name. It has special properties that make it effective against germs, viruses, and bacteria. It is a natural substance that even acts brutally on pathogens. Colloidal silver works even in conditions where the use of excessive antibiotics fails. It is known to soothe inflammation and aids in the faster recovery of wounds. Colloidal silver should however be administered under the careful observation of a natural medicine practitioner. Though it is a home remedy, it is advised to take complete information on dosage frequency.

Thus, we see that the treatment of diverticulitis does not necessarily have to be painful and expensive. With little care and effort, one can bring themselves out of the risk that the disease poses. Talking of all the measures undertaken, diet still plays a major role. The others will simply be instrumental in making the healing faster. The above methods, if adopted early can save a patient from the distress of a surgery.

Go on the Rest Mode

There is nothing more crucial than lending much-required rest to the body to heal up. Patients should not bother about being in bed all day long. This is what exactly is needed for the condition to become better. This is particularly true for milder forms of diverticulitis which are curable with the help of medications alone. There may arise absolutely no need for painful and cringe-worthy operations. Adequate rest would suffice.

Change the Diet

As discussed previously, diet is the major factor to control and cure diverticulitis. In the initial stages, it has to be solely rich in fluids and water. Gradually, it leads to taking in very few fibrous foods that are easy to digest. The intake of solid food may take some time until the intestines have fully recovered. Solid foods will restrict the smooth movement of food in the intestines, causing food to get stuck with its inability to pass out without restriction. The pressure thus applied may cause pouch formation leading to diverticulitis. Patients hence must be headstrong in adopting a whole new diet to cure themselves faster.

Incorporate Fresh Fruits and Vegetables in the Diet

Diverticulosis results from the lack of fiber and coarse grains in the diet. This is particularly true for fat-laden diets that provide little or no nutrition to the body. One must have at least three portions of fruits and vegetables in the entire day. The meal platter should also have greater portions of fruits, vegetables, and roughage that lend enough fiber to the body to ease out digestions and keep the digestive tract healthy. Fruits and vegetables are also potent in vitamins and other nutrients necessary to help bodily functions. Hence, a higher intake of fruits and vegetables will add to your overall health and not just for the cure of diverticulitis. The body will see improvement in overall activity and resistance against a wide variety of diseases.

Give Up on Red Meat

Red meat is the hard kind of meat that causes a variety of gastric problems. It is very difficult to digest and throws a lot of pressure on the intestines for grinding and absorption. Hence, it is very difficult to get it out of the system. Some say that red meat is not even fit for human consumption but well it is very much a part of diets around the world. Red meat has blood and high-fat content that in anyways not good for the human digestive system. The blood in the red meat may contain enzymes and bacteria that may spread infection in the gut thereby leading to digestive ailments that pile up to become diverticulitis. The high-fat content again causes low nutrient absorption problems. To cure diverticulitis, it may still be advised to eat softer meats like fish flesh, chicken, and other softer meats that are protein-rich and provide the body with nutrition.

Give Up on Alcohol

It is strongly advised that the patient either completely gives up on alcohol or at least keeps the intake under strict check. Alcohol disturbs the digestive function as much as it affects the liver. The functioning of both is closely linked and one directly affects the other. Bad quality or excessive alcohol may cause bacterial infection in the gut. Regular alcohol intake also causes dehydration that leads to the removal of water from the body. If this continues for long periods, it may cause problems of constipation and poor stomach health.

Keep Obesity Under Control

Obesity is the cause of major diseases in the human body. Excessive fat in the body makes people lethargic and drives them away from physical activity. Excess fat in the abdominal region also puts pressure on internal organs and causes digestion problems. People with high obesity usually are observed to have a high number of gastric problems. So it is really important to keep obesity under control through a combination of diet and exercise. This will also reflect positively on the other organs of the body and will improve psychological confidence also.

Drink More Fluids

Many overlook the importance of staying hydrated, but this tip may be the most effective in maintaining gut health. Drinking more fluids can help a high-fiber diet be moved even easier through the digestive process with fewer chances of obstructions developing. Keeping the fluid intake to a normal level is all that is needed. There doesn't seem to be much of a benefit for drinking excessive liquids during the day. Look to drink as many non-calorie beverages as you can with your diet each day which means no limits to water or tea.

The recommended water intake is generally:

- Men over 19 = 12 cups (about 3 liters) per day.
- Women over 19 = 9 cups (about 2 liters) per day.

Please contact your doctor to confirm that these values are okay for your specific scenario.

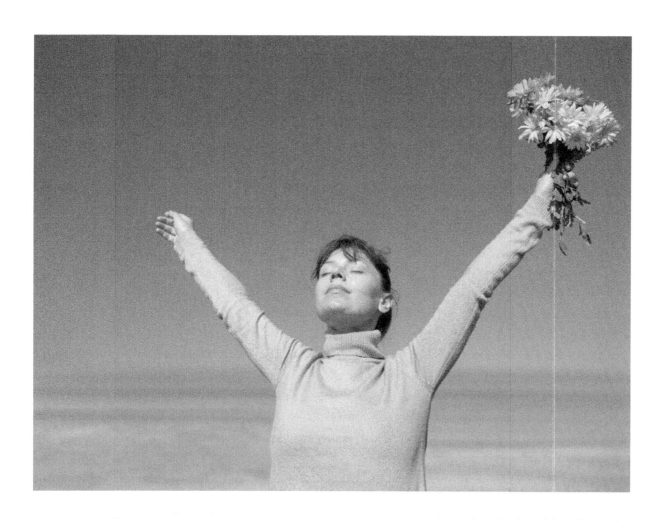

Chapter 4.   What foods are good for wellness.

It has been advised that a diet rich in fruits, vegetables, and whole grains is linked to a lower risk of diverticulitis.

Foods High in Fiber

A clear liquid diet has always been prescribed by doctors for persons suffering from severe diverticulitis flare-ups. After then, they may switch to a low-fiber diet until their symptoms improve. After a person's symptoms have improved, several sites suggest that they eat a high-fiber diet. Dietary fiber intake like 14 grams per 1,000 calories is recommended by the Dietary Guidelines for Americans, 2015-2020. Beans and pulses, like navy beans, chickpeas, split peas, and lentils; fruits, such as pear, avocado, apple, and prunes; vegetables, such as green peas, potatoes, squash, and parsnip; grains, such as bulgur, quinoa, barley, and whole wheat

Probiotics

The Probiotics are type of good bacteria that keep your gut healthy. Probiotics have been shown to be useful in treating symptomatic diverticular disease in a 2013 study, especially when paired with medicine and fermented foods including sauerkraut, kefir, tempeh, and miso.

People who have been taking antibiotics may also want to include these foods in their diet to help repopulate their gut with beneficial bacteria.

The possible probiotic effects of fermented foods, according to a 2019 review of the health benefits of fermented foods, can maintain a healthy digestive system and may relieve symptoms of irritable bowel syndrome (IBS). However, there isn't enough information to say whether or not they have an effect.

A normal Western diet is high in red meat and refined grains, with little fiber, and has been linked to an increased risk of diverticulitis, according to a 2017 study.

Nuts, popcorn, and seeds are safe for patients with diverticulitis, according to the USCF. Tomato, zucchini, cucumber, strawberry, and raspberry seeds are also safe to eat, according to experts. Doctors may also have previously advised people to remove these foods from their diets.

However, each person is very unique, and some people may discover that certain foods aggravate their symptoms. Anyone who discovers that a certain food causes discomfort or a change in symptoms should avoid it and consult their doctor or healthcare provider.

Foods high in FODMAPs

Fermentable oligosaccharides, disaccharides, monosaccharides, and polyols (FODMAP) is an acronym for fermentable oligosaccharides, disaccharides, monosaccharides, and polyols. These are carbohydrate items that have been linked to digestive issues like bloating, gas, and diarrhea, according to study.

According to a 2016 hypothesis, a high-fiber diet mixed with FODMAP foods may create excessive gas, which could exacerbate diverticulitis symptoms.

Onions, mushrooms, cauliflower, and garlic are examples of high FODMAP foods; apples, apricots, dried fruits, pears, and peaches are examples of high FODMAP foods; dairy foods, such as milk, yogurts, and cheeses; legumes and pulses are examples of high FODMAP foods; bread and cereals are examples of high FODMAP foods; sugars and sweeteners are examples of high FODMAP foods; and sugars and sweeteners are examples of high FOD

Because several of these foods also include helpful fiber, it's crucial to talk to a doctor about your meal choices and elimination. Because each person's dietary requirements and sensitivities are unique, doctors advise seeking professional advice.

Red meat.

Higher diets of red and processed meat have been associated to diverticulitis in studies. According to a reliable source from 2017, if people follow a healthy diet and lifestyle, they can lose weight. It's possible that half of all occurrences of diverticulitis may be avoided.

Here's an example of a one-day diverticulitis diet that's low in fiber and high in protein.

Breakfast

½ cup (89 grams) cream of wheat (0.5 grams of fiber)

one slice of white toast with margarine (1 gram of fiber)

three scrambled eggs.

Lunch

Two slices of white bread with butter (2 grams of fiber)

4 ounces (113 grams) of tuna

1 cup (240 grams) of chicken noodle soup (1 gram of fiber)

Snack

One cup (226 grams) of low-fat cottage cheese

Dinner

Four ounces (113 grams) of chicken breast

1 cup (174 grams) of white rice (0.5 grams of fiber)

½ cup (73 grams) of cooked green beans (2 grams of fiber)

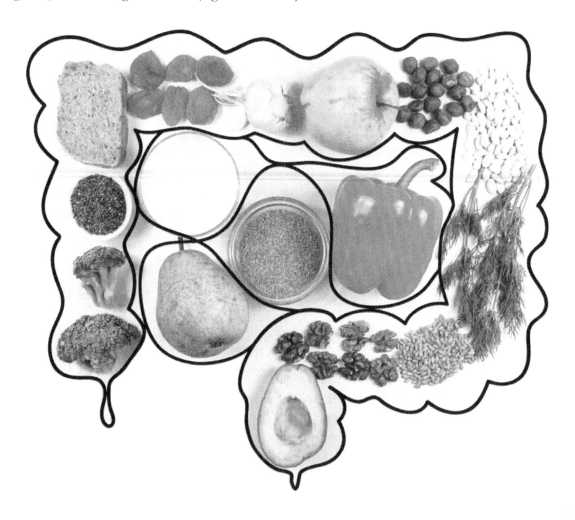

Chapter 5. A list of foods to avoid

According to experts, diet may or may not play a role in diverticulitis. Diverticulitis patients must avoid a few foods in particular. You'll notice that certain foods help or hurt your condition. If you have an acute case of diverticulitis, the doctor may advise you to cut back on the fiber intake for a while. They may advise you to avoid solid foods entirely and stick to a clear-liquid diet for a few days. This will allow your digestive system to rest. Then, your doctor may advise you to eat more high-fiber foods as your symptoms improve. In some studies, high-fiber diets have been linked to a lower risk of diverticulitis. Other studies have looked into the potential benefits of dietary or supplemental fiber for diverticular disease. However, the role fiber should play is still unknown. Limiting your intake of red meat, high-fat dairy products, and refined grain products may also be recommended by your doctor. According to a large cohort study, people who eat a diet high in these foods are more likely to develop diverticulitis than people who eat a diet high in fruits, vegetables, and whole grains. Diet can help you manage diverticulitis and your digestive health in general. Diverticulosis patients are usually advised to eat a high-fiber diet. Fruits and vegetables, whole grains, dried beans and lentils are all high in fiber. Previously, doctors advised people with diverticulosis to avoid nuts, popcorn, and seeds because these particles were thought to enter or block the diverticula. However, more recent research suggests that these foods are not harmful and may benefit some patients due to their high fiber content. Diverticulosis symptoms can vary from patient to patient, and some people may find that certain foods aggravate their symptoms. Below are seven low-fiber, high-sugar foods which may increase the risk of developing diverticulosis or trigger symptoms of diverticulosis:

Red meat

A new study published in Gut found that men who eat more red meat have a higher risk of developing diverticulitis. This is especially true if they eat unprocessed red meat. Regardless of fiber intake, a study found that red meat consumption was linked to a composite outcome of the symptomatic diverticular disease that included 385 incident cases over four years. Over 26 years, the researchers looked at the link between meat consumption-total red meat, unprocessed red meat, red, processed meat, poultry, and fish- and the risk of incident diverticulitis in 764 cases. According to the study, unprocessed red meat, not processed red meat, was the primary driver of the link between total red meat consumption and the risk of diverticulitis. Unprocessed meat (e.g., steak) is typically consumed in larger portions than processed meat, which may result in a larger indigestible piece in the large bowel and cause different variations in the colonic microbiota, as well as higher cooking temperatures used to prepare unprocessed meat, which may affect proinflammatory mediators in the colon or bacterial composition. Another reason to limit red meat consumption, according to new research, is that it puts you at a higher risk of developing the painful digestive disorder diverticulitis. Men who consumed red meat six or more times a week were fifty-eight percent more likely to develop it, according to a new 26-year study.

Fatty Foods

If you have been recently diagnosed with diverticulitis, you should avoid eating foods high in fat at all costs. Fried foods, like French fries, wings, potato chips, pizza, burgers, and anything else with high-fat content, fall into this category. Fatty foods boost the digestive tract, causing inflammation and activating the intestines' reflexes, part of the digestive system affected by diverticulitis. In addition, fatty foods can cause gas and diarrhea, which are common symptoms of diverticulitis. The typical Western diet is high in fat, sugar, and fiber but low in fiber. As a result, a person's risk of developing diverticulitis may increase. However, according to a 2017 study involving over 46,000 male participants, avoiding fatty foods might very well help prevent or reduce the symptoms of diverticulitis.

Some foods that we think are healthy are shockingly high in fat. A blueberry muffin may appear to be a healthy breakfast option, but it is cake and high in sugar and fat. A salad is a coleslaw. Even though it is made with carrots and cabbage, coleslaw is dressed in a high-fat mayonnaise dressing. Salami, like sausages, can quickly increase the fat and calories in your meal. The average egg yolk has 5.6 grams of fat.

Similarly, pizza has a lot of cheese on it. This dish's fat content can be extremely high. A 40g serving of granola with nuts contains 180 calories and 8.2 grams of fat, 1.8 grams of saturated fat. Grilled mackerel has 452 calories and 35.8 grams of fat, 8.2 grams of saturated fat. The garlic butter quickly increases the bread's calorie and fat content. As a result, it's critical to keep track of the amount of food you consume.

- **Alcohol**

Being diagnosed with diverticular disease does not mean you will die, but you must adhere to a diverticulitis diet. If you have diverticulosis or diverticulitis, the diet includes a list of foods you should eat or avoid. Doctors advise against drinking alcohol that it can be difficult for someone who has a problem with alcohol. Alcoholism is an addiction that causes a person to drink despite the negative consequences – both frequently and in unhealthy amounts. Alcohol has a major impact on the gastrointestinal tract, which many people are unaware of. These negative effects are amplified if you abuse alcohol because you drink more heavily and frequently. The passage of food through your intestine is slowed by alcohol. The development of diverticulosis has been linked to a decrease in motility in the lower intestine (rectosigmoid). According to studies, alcohol drinkers are also more likely to develop diverticulosis and diverticular bleeding. Diverticulosis and alcoholism are both chronic illnesses that require long-term treatment. Even if you feel fine, you should check your pipes if you drink alcohol and are over 50. According to a new study, drinking alcohol increases the risk of developing colon diverticulosis. At first, there are few symptoms. However, failing to keep an eye out for this could lead to more serious issues and pain in the future. According to the researchers, the more alcohol patients consume and the older they get, the more likely they develop diverticulosis. Patients' chances of developing a problem increased nearly twofold when they drank alcohol. If you are suffering from both, alcohol treatment programs can help you overcome your problems.

- **Carbonated drinks**

If the diverticula are inflamed, it is best to drink only natural water and avoid alcohol, carbonated and sweetened beverages. Anything carbonated must be avoided. The accumulation of gas is just about as painful as the disease. In addition, carbonated drinks should be avoided because they can cause bloating and gas, aggravating the symptoms of diverticulitis.

- **Spicy foods**

If you like spicy food, you should avoid adding it to the food if you have diverticulitis. Even in people who do not have digestive problems, spicy foods aggravate the digestive system. Because diverticulitis is a condition affecting the digestive tract (intestines), it's best to stay away from spicy foods. If you have diverticulitis, for example, chili powder should be avoided. Spicy foods could indeed irritate as well as inflame the digestive tract, resulting in diarrhea, vomiting, and other symptoms linked to diverticulitis. If you have diverticulitis, you should avoid eating peppers, especially the red and green varieties, just as you should avoid spicy foods. Peppers, especially red and green peppers, have a natural spice that may aggravate the symptoms of diverticulitis.

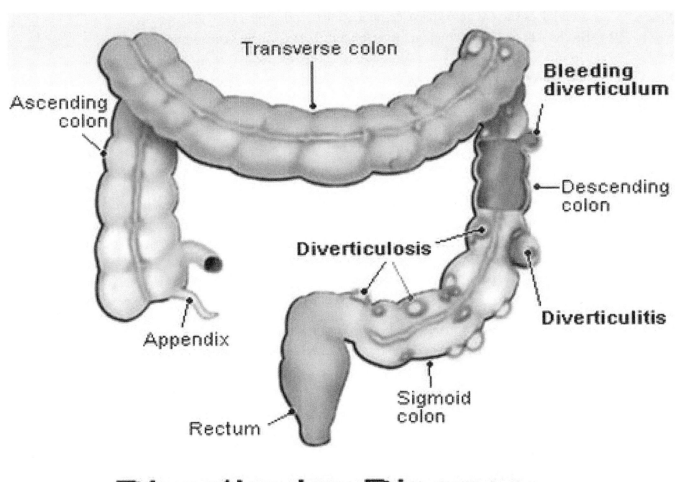

Diverticular Disease

Chapter 6.   Description of Recommended Dishes

Phase 1 – Clear Liquid Diet

When the patient experiences severe symptoms of diverticulitis, they should follow a clear liquid diet, which is called Phase 1 in the meal plan. The patient is required to consume only liquids without fiber to help in the healing process and strengthening of the colon.

Here is a list of foods that are permitted when one is following a clear liquid diet:

- Plain water
- Strained lemonade
- Clear sodas
- Fruit juices such as grape juice, cranberry juice, and apple juice.
- Broths – bone broth, bouillon, vegetable broth, and fat-free consommé.
- Gelatin
- Jelly – no seeds
- Coffee or tea without cream or milk
- Ice pops

Phase 2 – Low-Residue Diet

As soon as the liquid diet ends, the patient should consume a low-residue diet or a low-fiber diet. During Phase 2, you must limit your intake of fiber-rich foods for at least a week. The exact duration of this phase will depend on your condition and the advice of your physician.Here is a list of foods that are allowed and the foods that should be consumed thoughtfully.

- **Beverages –**

Coffee, decaf coffee, decaf tea, carbonated drinks, cocoa, and clear fruit drinks are allowed.
Alcoholic beverages or any beverages that contain pulp should be limited.

- **Cereals and bread –**

Light wheat or refined flour bread, soda crackers, and saltines are permitted. Cereals made with oats, rice, and wheat are also allowed.
Bread and rolls that contain fruits, nuts, and seeds are strictly prohibited. Patients are also recommended to avoid bread with whole grains, raisins, or bran. Corn bread and graham crackers should not be consumed.

- **Desserts –**

Desserts such as custards, plain puddings, tapioca, fruit whips, gelatin, fruit ice, smooth ice cream, yogurt, plain sherbet, cookies, and cakes can be consumed.
Cakes, puddings, or pastries containing nuts, raisins, seeds, dates, coconut, and fruits should not be eaten.

- **Eggs –**

Dishes made with eggs are allowed but must not contain any kind of nuts, seeds, or fruits.

- **Fruits and juices –**

Fruit juices that do not contain any pulp are allowed.

Canned products like applesauce, fruit cocktail, peaches, and cherries can be included in the diet.
Fresh fruits like bananas, grapefruit, cherries, nectarines, melons, plums, and peaches can also be consumed.
Fruits like pineapples, apples, pears, avocados, apricots, mangos, berries, pears, figs, dried dates, raisins, and prunes should be limited.

- **Cheese or butter –**

Cream cheese, American cheese, cottage cheese, Swiss or Monterey Jack cheese, cheddar cheese, and smooth peanut butter can be consumed.
Strong cheeses or those containing seeds should be avoided. Chunky peanut butter should not be consumed.

- **Meat –**

Tender, stewed, broiled, roast, or creamed beef, lamb, veal, ham, pork, fish, poultry, oysters, chopped clams, kidneys, and liver are allowed.
Patients should avoid fried meats, poultry, fish, highly seasoned meats, meats with whole spices, frankfurters, and sausages.

- **Soups –**

Soups made with pureed and creamed vegetables, strained vegetables, fish, or meat broths can be consumed.
Soups that contain seeds or vegetables or that are highly seasoned are not permitted in Phase 2.

- **Vegetables –**

Canned or cooked vegetables like asparagus, carrots, beets, artichoke hearts, greens, wax beans, chard, mushrooms, bean sprouts, pumpkin, and pimento can be consumed. Fresh or cooked tomatoes (avoid skin or seeds) can be a part of the diet as well.
Consumption of vegetables like cabbage, okra, summer squash, parsnips, rutabagas, broccoli, or corn should be avoided.

Phase 3 – High-Fiber Diet
As the patient transitions from Phase 2 (low-fiber diet) to Phase 3 (high-fiber diet), high-fiber foods should be gradually increased. A sudden increase in the fiber content can result in gas, diarrhea, or abdominal pain.
Some of the foods that contain high-fiber content and that can be included in the Phase 3 diet are:
- Legumes and beans
- Whole wheat bread
- Bran
- Whole grain cereals – oatmeal
- Wild rice and brown rice
- Fruits like bananas, pears, and apples
- Vegetables like corn, squash, carrots, and broccoli
- Whole wheat pasta and noodles

Chapter 7. Breakfast clear liquid

1. Apple Orange Juice

Preparation Time: 5 minutes
Cooking Time: 0 minutes
Servings: 2
Ingredients:

- 1 Gala apple, peeled, cored, and sliced
- 2 oranges, peeled, halved, and seeded
- 2 tsp. honey (optional)
- 3/4 cup water

Directions:

1. Squeeze each orange over a fine-mesh strainer.
2. Gently, press the pulp to extract as much liquid as possible.
3. Add in the apple, water, and orange juice in your blender and pulse.
4. Set a fine-mesh strainer in a bowl. Before transferring your juice into the strainer.
5. Once again, gently press the pulp to remove all possible liquid, then discard it.
6. Stir in your honey, then serve over ice.

Nutrition:

- Calories: 180 kcal
- Fat: 1 g
- Carbs: 43 g
- Fiber: 1 g
- Protein: 2 g

2. Pineapple Mint Juice

Preparation Time: 5 minutes.
Cooking Time: 0 minutes
Servings: 4
Ingredients:

- 3 cups pineapple, cored, sliced, and chunks
- 10–12 mint leaves, or to taste
- 2 tbsp. sugar, or to taste (optional)
- 1 ½ cup water
- 1 cup ice cubes

Directions:

1. Set all the ingredients into your blender, and pulse.
2. Set a fine-mesh strainer in a bowl. Before transferring your juice into the strainer.

3. Gently, press the pulp to extract all possible liquid, then discard it.
4. Serve over ice. Enjoy!

Nutrition:

- Calories: 78 kcal
- Fat: 1 g
- Carbs: 22 g
- Fiber: 2 g
- Protein: 1 g

3. Celery Apple Juice

Preparation Time: 5 minutes
Cooking Time: 0 minutes
Servings: 2
Ingredients:

- 12 celery stalks, peeled and chopped
- 3 Apple, peeled, cored, seeded, and sliced
- 1-inch ginger root, peeled and chopped
- 1/4 lemon juice
- 2 cups water

Directions:

1. Set all the ingredients into your blender, and pulse.
2. Set a fine-mesh strainer in a bowl. Before transferring your juice into the strainer.
3. Gently, press the pulp to extract all possible liquid, then discard it.
4. Serve over ice. Enjoy!

Nutrition:

- Calories: 119 kcal
- Fat: 1 g
- Carbs: 29 g
- Fiber: 7 g
- Protein: 2 g

4. Homemade Banana Apple Juice

Preparation Time: 10 minutes
Cooking Time: 0 minutes
Servings: 2
Ingredients:

- 2 bananas, peeled and sliced
- 1/2 apple, peeled, cored, and chopped
- 1 tbsp. honey
- 1 ½ cup water

Directions:

1. Set all the ingredients into your blender, and pulse.
2. Set a fine-mesh strainer in a bowl. Before transferring your juice into the strainer.
3. Gently, press the pulp to extract all possible liquid, then discard it.
4. Serve over ice. Enjoy!

Nutrition:
- Calories: 132 kcal
- Fat: 2 g
- Carbs: 27 g
- Fiber: 3 g
- Protein: 4 g

5.   Sweet Detox Juice

Preparation Time: 10 minutes
Cooking Time: 0 minutes
Servings: 2
Ingredients:
- 2 cups baby spinach, chopped
- 1 handful parsley, chopped
- 1 green apple, peeled, cored, seeded, and sliced
- 1 large English cucumber, seeded and chopped
- 1-inch ginger, peeled
- 1 lemon, juiced

Directions:
1. Set all the ingredients into your blender, and pulse.
2. Set a fine-mesh strainer in a bowl. Before transferring your juice into the strainer.
3. Gently, press the pulp to extract all possible liquid, then discard it.
4. Serve over ice. Enjoy!

Nutrition:
- Calories: 209 kcal
- Fat: 2 g
- Carbs: 48 g
- Fiber: 17 g
- Protein: 12 g

6.   Pineapple Ginger Juice

Preparation Time: 35 minutes
Cooking Time: 0 minutes
Servings: 7 cups
Ingredients:

- 10 cups pineapple, chopped
- 6 cups water
- 3 Fuji apples, chopped
- 4-inch ginger root, peeled and chopped
- 1/4 cup lemon juice
- 1/4 cup sugar

Directions:
1. Set all the ingredients into your blender, and pulse.
2. Set a fine-mesh strainer in a bowl. Before transferring your juice into the strainer.
3. Gently, press the pulp to extract all possible liquid, then discard it.
4. Serve over ice. Enjoy!

Nutrition:
- Calories: 71 kcal
- Fat: 1 g
- Carbs: 20 g
- Fiber: 3 g
- Protein: 1 g

7.   Carrot Orange Juice

Preparation Time: 15 minutes
Cooking Time: 0 minutes
Servings: 2
Ingredients:
- 1 medium yellow tomato, cut into wedges
- 1 orange, peeled and quartered
- 1 apple, peeled, cored, and chopped
- 4 jumbo carrots, peeled and chopped
- 2 cups water

Directions:
1. Set all the ingredients into your blender, and pulse.
2. Set a fine-mesh strainer in a bowl. Before transferring your juice into the strainer.
3. Gently, press the pulp to extract all possible liquid, then discard it.
4. Serve over ice. Enjoy!

Nutrition:
- Calories: 111 kcal
- Fat: 1 g
- Carbs: 24 g
- Fiber: 1 g
- Protein: 2 g

8. Strawberry Apple Juice

Preparation Time: 5 minutes
Cooking Time: 0 minutes
Servings: 8–10 ounces
Ingredients:

- 2 cups strawberries (tops removed)
- 1 red apple, peeled, seeded, cored, and chopped
- 1 tbsp. chia seeds
- 1 cup water

Directions:

1. Set all the ingredients into your blender, and pulse.
2. Set a fine-mesh strainer in a bowl. Before transferring your juice into the strainer.
3. Gently, press the pulp to extract all possible liquid, then discard it.
4. Add in your chia seeds, then leave to sit for at least 5 minutes.
5. Serve over ice. Enjoy!

Nutrition:

- Calories: 245 kcal
- Fat: 5 g
- Carbs: 52 g
- Fiber: 7 g
- Protein: 4 g

9. Autumn Energizer Juice

Preparation Time: 10 minutes
Cooking Time: 0 minutes
Servings: 2
Ingredients:

- 2 pears, peeled, seeded, and chopped
- 2 Ambrosia apples, peeled, cored, and chopped
- 2 Granny Smith apples, peeled, cored, chopped
- 2 mandarins, juiced
- 2 cups sweet potato, peeled and chopped
- 1-pint cape gooseberries
- 2 inches ginger root, peeled

Directions:

1. Set all the ingredients into your blender, and pulse.
2. Set a fine-mesh strainer in a bowl. Before transferring your juice into the strainer.

3. Gently, press the pulp to extract all possible liquid, then discard it.
4. Serve over ice. Enjoy!

Nutrition:

- Calories: 170 kcal
- Fat: 3 g
- Carbs: 33 g
- Fiber: 9 g
- Protein: 4 g

10. Asian Inspired Wonton Broth

Preparation Time: 5 minutes
Cooking Time: 15 minutes
Servings: 2
Ingredients:

- 1 chicken thigh, skin on
- 1 carrot, coarsely chopped
- 1 celery stalk, coarsely chopped
- 1 small onion, quartered
- 3 dime-sized ginger pieces
- 2 tbsp. kosher salt
- 1/4 tsp. turmeric
- 1/8 tsp. MSG (don't leave it out)
- 5 white peppercorns (can be substituted with black)
- 1-liter water

Directions:

1. Transfer all the ingredients to your stockpot. Top with enough water to cover then allow to come to a boil on high heat slowly.
2. Switch to low heat and simmer for at least 15 minutes.
3. Set and pour the mixture through a fine-mesh strainer into a large bowl.
4. Taste and season with salt.
5. Serve hot.

Nutrition:

- Calories: 181 kcal
- Fat: 7 g
- Carbs: 14 g
- Fiber: 1 g
- Protein: 14 g

11. Mushroom, Cauliflower and Cabbage Broth

Preparation Time: 10 minutes

Cooking Time: 15 minutes
Servings: 2
Ingredients:

- 1 large yellow onion
- 1 cup celery stalks, chopped
- 2 carrots, diced or cubed
- 10 French beans
- 1/2 cabbage, diced
- 1–2 stalks celery leaves
- 1 ½ cup mushrooms, sliced
- 8 florets cauliflower
- 1 tsp. garlic, chopped
- 1 tsp. ginger, chopped
- 1 tbsp. oil
- 1 scallion stalk
- 1/2 tsp. pepper, crushed

Directions:

1. Transfer all the ingredients to your stockpot. Top with enough water to cover, then allow to come to a boil on high heat slowly.
2. Switch to low heat and simmer for 15 minutes.
3. Set and pour the mixture through a fine-mesh strainer into a large bowl. Mash the vegetables well to extract all their juices.
4. Taste and season with salt. Enjoy.

Nutrition:

- Calories: 141 kcal
- Fat: 5 g
- Carbs: 22 g
- Fiber: 7 g
- Protein: 5 g

12. Indian Inspired Vegetable Stock

Preparation Time: 10 minutes
Cooking Time: 11 minutes
Servings: 3
Ingredients:

- 3/4 cup onions, roughly chopped
- 3/4 cup carrot, roughly chopped
- 3/4 cup tomatoes, roughly chopped
- 3/4 cup potatoes, roughly chopped
- 1 tsp. turmeric
- Salt to taste

Directions:

1. Transfer all the ingredients to your stockpot. Top with enough water to cover, then allow to come to a boil on high heat slowly.
2. Switch to low heat and simmer for 11 minutes.
3. Set and pour the mixture through a fine-mesh strainer into a large bowl. Taste and season with salt.
4. Serve hot. Enjoy!

Nutrition:

- Calories: 103 kcal
- Fat: 0.2 mg
- Carbs: 23.3 g
- Fiber: 3.1 g
- Protein: 2.2 g

13. Beef Bone Broth

Preparation Time: 10 minutes
Cooking Time: 15 minutes
Servings: 8
Ingredients:

- 2 pounds beef bones
- 1 onion, chopped in quarters
- 2 celery stalks, chopped in half
- 2 carrots, chopped in half
- 3 whole garlic cloves
- 2 bay leaves
- 1 tbsp. salt
- Filtered water (enough to cover bones)

Directions:

1. Transfer the bones and vegetables to your stockpot. Top with enough water to cover, then allow to come to a boil on high heat slowly.
2. Switch to low heat and simmer for at least 15 minutes.
3. Set and pour the mixture through a fine-mesh strainer into a large bowl. Taste and season with salt.
4. Serve hot.

Nutrition:

- Calories: 69 kcal
- Fat: 4 g
- Carbs: 1 g
- Fiber: 0.1 g
- Protein: 6 g

14. Ginger, Mushroom and Cauliflower Broth

Preparation Time: 10 minutes
Cooking Time: 15 minutes
Servings: 3
Ingredients:

- 1 large yellow onion
- 1 cup celery stalks, chopped
- 2 carrots, diced or cubed
- 10 French beans
- 1 ginger root, peeled, diced, or grated
- 1–2 stalks celery leaves or coriander leaves
- 1 ½ cup mushrooms, sliced
- 8 florets cauliflower
- 1 tsp. garlic, chopped
- 1 tbsp. oil
- 1 stalk spring onion greens or scallions
- 1/2 tsp. crushed pepper or ground pepper

Directions:

1. Transfer all the ingredients to your stockpot. Top with enough water to cover, then allow to come to a boil on high heat slowly.
2. Switch to low heat and simmer for at least 15 minutes.
3. Set and pour the mixture through a fine-mesh strainer into a large bowl. Taste and season with salt.
4. Serve hot. Enjoy!

Nutrition:

- Calories: 141 kcal
- Fat: 5 g
- Carbs: 22 g
- Fiber: 7 g
- Protein: 5 g

15. Fish Broth

Preparation Time: 15 minutes
Cooking Time: 15 minutes
Servings: 3
Ingredients:

- 1 large onion, chopped
- 1 large carrot chopped
- 1 fennel bulb and fronds, chopped (optional)
- 3 celery stalks, chopped
- Salt

- 2–5 pounds fish bones and heads
- 1 handful dried mushrooms (optional)
- 2–4 bay leaves
- 1-star anise pod (optional)
- 1–2 tsp. thyme, dried or fresh
- 3–4 pieces dried kombu kelp (optional)

Directions:

1. Transfer the bones and vegetables to your stockpot. Top with enough water to cover, then allow to come to a boil on high heat slowly.
2. Set to low heat and simmer for 45 minutes.
3. Set and pour the mixture through a fine-mesh strainer into a large bowl. Taste and season with salt.
4. Serve hot. Enjoy!

Nutrition:

- Calories: 29 kcal
- Fat: 1 g
- Carbs: 2 g
- Fiber: 1 g
- Protein: 1 g

16. Clear Pumpkin Broth

Preparation Time: 15 minutes
Cooking Time: 15 minutes
Servings: 6
Ingredients:

- 6 cups water
- 2 tbsp. ginger, minced
- 2 cups potatoes, peeled and diced
- 3 cups kabocha, peeled and diced
- 1 carrot, peeled and diced
- 1 onion, diced
- 1/2 cup scallions, chopped

Directions:

1. Transfer the bones and vegetables to your stockpot. Top with enough water to cover, then allow to come to a boil on high heat slowly.
2. Switch to low heat and simmer for at least 15 minutes.
3. Set and pour the mixture through a fine-mesh strainer into a large bowl. Taste and season with salt.
4. Serve hot. Enjoy!

Nutrition:

- Calories: 216 kcal
- Fat: 1 g

- Carbs: 37 g
- Fiber: 4 g
- Protein: 8 g

17.   Healthier Apple Juice
Preparation Time: 5 minutes
Cooking Time: 0 minutes
Servings: 2
Ingredients:
- 8 medium apples, cored and quartered

Directions:
1.   Add the apples into a juicer and extract the juice according to the manufacturer's method.
2.   Through a cheesecloth-lined sieve, strain the juice and transfer it into 2 glasses.
3.   Serve immediately.

Nutrition:
- Calories: 164 kcal
- Carbs: 123.6 g
- Protein: 2.4 g
- Fat: 1.6 g
- Sugar: 90 g
- Sodium: 123 mg
- Fiber: 21.6 g

18.   Citrus Apple Juice
Preparation Time: 5 minutes
Cooking Time: 0 minutes
Servings: 2
Ingredients:
- 5 large apples, cored and chopped
- 1 small lemon
- 1 cup fresh orange juice

Directions:
1.   Attach all the ingredients in a blender and pulse until well combined.
2.   Through a cheesecloth-lined sieve, strain the juice and transfer it into 2 glasses.
3.   Serve immediately.

Nutrition:
- Calories: 148 kcal
- Carbs: 90.6 g
- Protein: 2.4 g
- Fat: 1.3 g
- Sugar: 68.6g
- Sodium: 6 mg

- Fiber: 14 g

19.   Richly Fruity Juice
Preparation Time: 15 minutes
Cooking Time: 10 minutes
Servings: 2
Ingredients:
- 5 large green apples, cored and sliced
- 2 cups seedless white grapes
- 2 tsp. fresh lime juice

Directions:
1.   Set all ingredients into a juicer and extract the juice according to the manufacturer's method.
2.   Through a cheesecloth-lined sieve, strain the juice and transfer it into 2 glasses.
3.   Serve immediately.

Nutrition:
- Calories: 152 kcal
- Carbs: 92.8 g
- Protein: 2.1 g
- Fat: 1.3 g
- Sugar: 73 g
- Sodium: 7 mg
- Fiber: 14.3 g

20.   Delicious Grape Juice
Preparation Time: 15 minutes
Cooking Time: 0 minutes
Servings: 3
Ingredients:
- 2 cups white seedless grapes
- 1 ½ cup filtered water
- 6–8 ice cubes

Directions:
1.   Attach all the ingredients in a blender and pulse until well combined.
2.   Through a cheesecloth-lined sieve, strain the juice and transfer it into 3 glasses.
3.   Serve immediately.

Nutrition:
- Calories: 41 kcal
- Carbs: 10.5 g
- Protein: 0.4 g
- Fat: 0.2 g
- Sugar: 10 g
- Sodium: 1 mg

- Fiber: 10 g

21. Lemony Grape Juice

Preparation Time: 15 minutes
Cooking Time: 0 minutes
Servings: 3
Ingredients:
- 4 cups seedless white grapes
- 2 tbsp. fresh lemon juice

Directions:
1. Attach all the ingredients in a blender and pulse until well combined.
2. Through a cheesecloth-lined sieve, strain the juice and transfer it into 3 glasses.
3. Serve immediately.

Nutrition:
- Calories: 85 kcal
- Carbs: 21.3 g
- Protein: 0.9 g
- Fat: 0.5 g
- Sugar: 20.1 g
- Sodium: 4 mg
- Fiber: 1.1 g

22. Holiday Special Juice

Preparation Time: 15 minutes
Cooking Time: 0 minutes
Servings: 4
Ingredients:
- 4 cups fresh cranberries
- 1 tbsp. fresh lemon juice
- 2 cups filtered water
- 1 tsp. raw honey

Directions:
1. Attach all the ingredients in a blender and pulse until well combined.
2. Through a cheesecloth-lined sieve, strain the juice and transfer it into 4 glasses.
3. Serve immediately.

Nutrition:
- Calories: 66 kcal
- Carbs: 11.5 g
- Protein: 0 g
- Fat: 0 g
- Sugar: 5.5 g
- Sodium: 1 mg

- Fiber: 4 g

23. Vitamin C Rich Juice

Preparation Time: 15 minutes
Cooking Time: 0 minutes
Servings: 2
Ingredients:
- 8 oranges, peeled and sectioned

Directions:
1. Add the orange sections into a juicer and extract the juice according to the manufacturer's method.
2. Through a cheesecloth-lined sieve, strain the juice and transfer it into 2 glasses.
3. Serve immediately.

Nutrition:
- Calories: 146 kcal
- Carbs: 86.5 g
- Protein: 6.9 g
- Fat: 0.9 g
- Sugar: 68.8 g
- Sodium: 0 mg
- Fiber: 17.7 g

24. Incredible Fresh Juice

Preparation Time: 15 minutes
Cooking Time: 0 minutes
Servings: 4
Ingredients:
- 2 pounds carrots, trimmed and scrubbed
- 6 small oranges, peeled and sectioned

Directions:
1. Add the carrots and orange sections into a juicer and extract the juice according to the manufacturer's method.
2. Through a cheesecloth-lined sieve, strain the juice and transfer it into 4 glasses.
3. Serve immediately.

Nutrition:
- Calories: 183 kcal
- Carbs: 44.9 g
- Protein: 3.7 g
- Fat: 0.2 g
- Sugar: 29.1 g
- Sodium: 156 mg
- Fiber: 10.2 g

25. Favorite Summer Lemonade

Preparation Time: 15 minutes
Cooking Time: 0 minutes
Servings: 8
Ingredients:
- 8 cups filtered water
- 1/2 cup fresh lemon juice
- 1/4 tsp. pure stevia extract
- Ice cubes, as required

Directions:
1. In a pitcher, place the water, lemon juice, and stevia. Mix well.
2. Through a cheesecloth-lined sieve, strain the lemonade in another pitcher.
3. Refrigerate for 30–40 minutes.
4. Set ice cubes in serving glasses and fill with lemonade.
5. Serve chilled.

Nutrition:
- Calories: 4 kcal
- Carbs: 0.3 g
- Protein: 0.1 g
- Fat: 0.1 g
- Sugar: 0.3 g
- Sodium: 3 mg
- Fiber: 0.1 g

26. Ultimate Fruity Punch

Preparation Time: 15 minutes
Cooking Time: 0 minutes
Servings: 12
Ingredients:
- 3 cups fresh pineapple juice
- 2 cups fresh orange juice
- 1 cup fresh ruby red grapefruit juice
- 1/4 cup fresh lime juice
- 2 cups seedless watermelon, cut into bite-sized chunks
- 2 cups fresh pineapple, cut into bite-sized chunks
- 2 oranges, peeled and cut into wedges
- 2 limes, quartered
- 1 lemon, sliced
- 2 (12 ounces) cans diet lemon-lime soda
- Crushed ice, as required

Directions:
1. In a large pitcher, add all ingredients except for soda cans and ice. Stir to combine.
2. Set aside for 30 minutes.
3. Through a cheesecloth-lined sieve, strain the punch into another large pitcher.
4. Set the glasses with ice and top with punch about 3/4 of the mixture.
5. Add a splash of the soda and serve.

Nutrition:
- Calories: 95 kcal
- Carbs: 23.4 g
- Protein: 1.3 g
- Fat: 0.3 g
- Sugar: 18.3 g
- Sodium: 152 mg
- Fiber: 1.8 g

27. Thirst Quencher Sports Drink

Preparation Time: 15 minutes
Cooking Time: 0 minutes
Servings: 8
Ingredients:
- 7 cups spring water
- 1 cup fresh apple juice
- 2–3 tsp. fresh lime juice
- 2 tbsp. honey
- 1/4 tsp. sea salt

Directions:
1. In a large pitcher, add all ingredients and stir to combine.
2. Through a cheesecloth-lined sieve, strain the punch into another large pitcher.
3. Refrigerate to chill before serving.

Nutrition:
- Calories: 30 kcal
- Carbs: 7.8 g
- Protein: 0.1 g
- Fat: 0 g
- Sugar: 7.3 g
- Sodium: 60 mg
- Fiber: 0.1 g

28. Refreshing Sports Drink

Preparation Time: 15 minutes

Cooking Time: 0 minutes
Servings: 9
Ingredients:

- 8 cups fresh cold water, divided
- 3/4 cup fresh orange juice
- 1/4 cup fresh lemon juice
- 1/4 cup fresh limes juice
- 3 tbsp. honey
- 1/2 tsp. salt

Directions:

1. In a large pitcher, add all ingredients and stir to combine.
2. Through a cheesecloth-lined sieve, strain the punch into another large pitcher.
3. Refrigerate to chill before serving.

Nutrition:

- Calories: 33 kcal
- Carbs: 8.1 g
- Protein: 0.2 g
- Fat: 0.1 g
- Sugar: 7.6 g
- Sodium: 130 mg
- Fiber: 0.1 g

29. Perfect Sunny Day Tea

Preparation Time: 15 minutes
Cooking Time: 3 minutes
Servings: 6
Ingredients:

- 5 cups filtered water
- 5 green tea bags
- 1/4 cup fresh lemon juice, strained
- 1/4 cup fresh lime juice, strained
- 1/4 cup honey
- Ice cubes, as required

Directions:

1. In a medium pan, add 2 cups of water and bring to a boil.
2. Set in the tea bags and turn off the heat.
3. Immediately, cover the pan and steep for 3–4 minutes.
4. With a large spoon, gently press the tea bags against the pan to extract the tea completely.
5. Detach the tea bags from the pan and discard them.
6. Set honey and stir until dissolved.

7. In a large pitcher, place the tea, lemon, and lime juice and stir to combine.
8. Add the remaining cold water and stir to combine.
9. Refrigerate to chill before serving.
10. Attach ice cubes in serving glasses and fill with tea.
11. Serve chilled.

Nutrition:

- Calories: 46 kcal
- Carbs: 12 g
- Protein: 0.1 g
- Fat: 0.1 g
- Sugar: 11.8 g
- Sodium: 3 mg
- Fiber: 0.1 g

30. Nutritious Green Tea

Preparation Time: 15 minutes
Cooking Time: 4 minutes
Servings: 4
Ingredients:

- 4 cups filtered water
- 4 orange peel strips
- 4 lemon peel strips
- 4 green tea bags
- 2 tsp. honey

Directions:

1. In a medium pan, add the water, orange, and lemon peel strips over medium-high heat and bring to a boil.
2. Set the heat to low and stir, uncovered, for about 10 minutes.
3. With a slotted spoon, remove the orange and lemon peel strips and discard them.
4. Attach in the tea bags and turn off the heat.
5. Immediately, cover the pan and steep for 3 minutes.
6. With a large spoon, gently press the tea bags against the pan to extract the tea completely.
7. Detach the tea bags from the pan and discard them.
8. Add honey and stir until dissolved.
9. Strain the tea in mugs and serve immediately.

Nutrition:

- Calories: 11 kcal
- Carbs: 3 g

- Protein: 0 g
- Fat: 0 g
- Sugar: 2.9 g
- Sodium: 0 mg
- Fiber: 0.1 g

31.   Simple Black Tea

Preparation Time: 10 minutes
Cooking Time: 3 minutes
Servings: 2
Ingredients:
- 2 cups filtered water
- 1/2 tsp. black tea leaves
- 1 tsp. honey

Directions:
1.   In a pan, add the water and bring to a boil.
2.   Stir in the tea leaves and turn off the heat.
3.   Immediately, cover the pan and steep for 3 minutes.
4.   Add honey and stir until dissolved.
5.   Strain the tea in mugs and serve immediately.

Nutrition:
- Calories: 11 kcal
- Carbs: 2.9 g
- Protein: 0 g
- Fat: 0 g
- Sugar: 2.9 g
- Sodium: 123 mg
- Fiber: 0 g

32.   Lemony Black Tea

Preparation Time: 10 minutes
Cooking Time: 3 minutes
Servings: 6
Ingredients:
- 1 tbsp. black tea leaves
- 1 lemon, sliced thinly
- 1 cinnamon stick
- 6 cups boiling water

Directions:
1.   In a large teapot, place the tea leaves, lemon slices, and cinnamon stick.
2.   Pour hot water over the ingredients and immediately cover the teapot.
3.   Set aside for about 5 minutes to steep.

4.   Strain the tea in mugs and serve immediately.

Nutrition:
- Calories: 1
- Carbs: 0.2 g
- Protein: 0 g
- Fat: 0 g
- Sugar: 0.1 g
- Sodium: 0 mg
- Fiber: 0.1 g

33.   Metabolism Booster Coffee

Preparation Time: 5 minutes
Cooking Time: 4 minutes
Servings: 1
Ingredients:
- 1/4 tsp. coffee powder
- 1 ¼ cup filtered water
- 1 tsp. fresh lemon juice
- 1 tsp. honey

Directions:
1.   In a small pan, attach the water and coffee powder. Bring it to boil.
2.   Cook for about 1 minute.
3.   Detach from the heat and pour into a serving mug.
4.   Add the honey and lemon juice, then stir until dissolved
5.   Serve hot.

Nutrition:
- Calories: 23 kcal
- Carbs: 6 g
- Protein: 0.1 g
- Fat: 0 g
- Sugar: 5.9 g
- Sodium: 1 mg
- Fiber: 0 g

34.   Best Homemade Broth

Preparation Time: 15 minutes
Cooking Time: 15 minutes
Servings: 8
Ingredients:
- 1 (3 pounds) chicken, cut into pieces
- 5 medium carrots
- 4 celery stalks with leaves

- 6 fresh thyme sprigs
- 6 fresh parsley sprigs
- Salt to taste
- 9 cups cold water

Directions:
1. In a large pan, attach all the ingredients over medium-high heat and bring to a boil.
2. Set the heat to medium-low and stir, covered for about 15 minutes, occasionally skimming the foam from the surface.
3. Through a fine-mesh sieve, strain the broth into a large bowl.
4. Serve hot.

Nutrition:
- Calories: 275 kcal
- Carbs: 4.3 g
- Protein: 49.7 g
- Fat: 5.2 g
- Sugar: 2 g
- Sodium: 160 mg
- Fiber: 1.2 g

35. Clean Testing Broth

Preparation Time: 5 hours 50 minutes
Cooking Time: 15 minutes
Servings: 10
Ingredients:
- 4 pounds chicken bones
- Salt to taste
- 10 cups filtered water
- 2 tbsp. apple cider vinegar
- 1 lemon, quartered
- 3 bay leaves
- 3 tsp. ground turmeric
- 2 tbsp. peppercorns

Directions:
1. Preheat the oven to 400°F.
2. Arrange the bones onto a large baking sheet and sprinkle with salt.
3. Roast for about 45 minutes.
4. Detach from the oven and transfer the bones into a large pan.
5. Add the remaining ingredients and stir to combine.
6. Put the pan over medium-high heat and bring to a boil.

7. Set the heat to low and stir, covered for about 4–5 hours, occasionally skimming the foam from the surface.
8. Through a fine-mesh sieve, strain the broth into a large bowl.
9. Serve hot.

Nutrition:
- Calories: 140 kcal
- Carbs: 0.6 g
- Protein: 25 g
- Fat: 2.6 g
- Sugar: 0.1 g
- Sodium: 73 mg
- Fiber: 0.1 g

36. Healing Broth

Preparation Time: 10 hours 25 minutes
Cooking Time: 15 minutes
Servings: 12
Ingredients:
- 3 tbsp. extra-virgin olive oil
- 2 ½ pounds chicken bones
- 4 celery stalks, chopped roughly
- 3 large carrots, peeled and chopped roughly
- 1 bay leaf
- 1 tbsp. black peppercorns
- 2 whole cloves
- 1 tbsp. apple cider vinegar
- Warm water, as required

Directions:
1. In a Dutch oven, heat the oil over medium-high heat and sear the bones for about 3–5 minutes or until browned.
2. With a slotted spoon, transfer the bones into a bowl.
3. In the same pan, add the celery stalks and carrots. Cook for about 15 minutes, stirring occasionally.
4. Add browned bones, bay leaf, black peppercorns, cloves, and vinegar. Stir to combine.
5. Add enough warm water to cover the bones mixture completely and bring to a gentle boil.
6. Set the heat to low and stir, covered for about 8–10 hours, occasionally skimming the foam from the surface.
7. Through a fine-mesh sieve, strain the broth into a large bowl.
8. Serve hot.

Nutrition:
- Calories: 67 kcal
- Carbs: 2 g
- Protein: 5.7 g
- Fat: 4.1 g
- Sugar: 1 g
- Sodium: 29 mg
- Fiber: 0.5 g

37. Veggie Lover's Broth

Preparation Time: 2 hours 5 minutes
Cooking Time: 15 minutes
Servings: 10
Ingredients:
- 4 carrots, peeled and chopped roughly
- 4 celery stalks, chopped roughly
- 3 parsnips, peeled and chopped roughly
- 2 large potatoes, peeled and chopped roughly
- 1 medium beet, trimmed and chopped roughly
- 1 large bunch fresh parsley
- 1 (1 inch) piece fresh ginger, sliced
- Filtered water, as required

Directions:
1. In a pan, add all the ingredients over medium-high heat.
2. Add enough water to cover the veggie mixture and bring to a boil.
3. Set the heat to low and simmer, covered for about 2–3 hours.
4. Through a fine-mesh sieve, strain the broth into a large bowl.
5. Serve hot.

Nutrition:
- Calories: 82 kcal
- Carbs: 19 g
- Protein: 1.9 g
- Fat: 0.2 g
- Sugar: 3.9 g
- Sodium: 37 mg
- Fiber: 3.7 g

38. Brain Healthy Broth

Preparation Time: 12 hours 5 minutes
Cooking Time: 10 minutes

Servings: 6
Ingredients:
- 12 cups filtered water
- 2 pounds non-oily fish heads and bones
- 1/4 cup apple cider vinegar
- Sea salt to taste

Directions:
1. In a large pan, attach all the ingredients over medium-high heat.
2. Add enough water to cover the veggie mixture and bring to a boil.
3. Set the heat to low and simmer, covered for about 15 minutes, occasionally skimming the foam from the surface.
4. Through a fine-mesh sieve, strain the broth into a large bowl.
5. Serve hot.

Nutrition:
- Calories: 75 kcal
- Carbs: 0.1 g
- Protein: 13.4 g
- Fat: 1.7 g
- Sugar: 0 g
- Sodium: 253 mg
- Fiber: 0 g

39. Minerals Rich Broth

Preparation Time: 15 minutes
Cooking Time: 15 minutes
Servings: 8
Ingredients:
- 5–7 pounds non-oily fish carcasses and heads
- 2 tbsp. olive oil
- 3 carrots, scrubbed and chopped roughly
- 2 celery stalks, chopped roughly

Directions:
1. In a pan, heat the oil over medium-low heat and cook the carrots and celery for about 20 minutes, stirring occasionally.
2. Add the fish bones and enough water to cover by 1-inch and stir to combine.
3. Set the heat to medium-high and bring to a boil.
4. Set the heat to low, cover, and cook for about 1–2 hours, occasionally skimming the foam from the surface.

5.   Through a fine-mesh sieve, strain the broth into a large bowl.
6.   Serve hot.
Nutrition:
- Calories: 113 kcal
- Carbs: 2.5 g
- Protein: 13.7 g
- Fat: 5.2 g
- Sugar: 1.2 g
- Sodium: 234 mg
- Fiber: 0.7 g

40.   Holiday Favorite Gelatin
Preparation Time: 15 minutes
Cooking Time: 15 minutes
Servings: 6
Ingredients:
- 1 tbsp. grass-fed gelatin powder
- 1 ¾ cup fresh apple juice, warmed
- 1/4 cup boiling water
- 1–2 drops fresh lemon juice
Directions:
1.   In a medium bowl, pour in the tbsp. of gelatin powder.
2.   Add just enough warm apple juice to cover the gelatin and stir well.
3.   Set aside for about 2–3 minutes or until it forms a thick syrup.
4.   Add 1/4 cup of the boiling water and stir until gelatin is dissolved completely.
5.   Add the remaining juice and lemon juice then stir well.
6.   Transfer the mixture into a parchment paper-lined baking dish and refrigerate for 2 hours or until the top is firm before serving.
Nutrition:
- Calories: 40 kcal
- Carbs: 8.2 g
- Protein: 1.9 g
- Fat: 0.1 g

- Sugar: 7 g
- Sodium: 5 mg
- Fiber: 0.2 g

41.   Chicken Bone Broth
Preparation Time: 10 minutes
Cooking Time: 15 minutes
Servings: 8
Ingredients:
- 3–4 pounds bones (from 1 chicken)
- 4 cups water
- 2 large carrots, cut into chunks
- 2 large stalks celery
- 1 large onion
- 2 cups Fresh rosemary sprigs
- 3 fresh thyme sprigs
- 2 tbsp. apple cider vinegar
- 1 tsp. kosher salt
Directions:
1.   Put all the ingredients in your pot and allow to sit for 10 minutes.
2.   Pressure cook and adjust the time to 15 minutes.
3.   Set the release naturally until the float valve drops and then unlock the lid.
4.   Strain the broth and transfer it into a storage container. The broth can be refrigerated for 3–5 days or frozen for up to 6 months.
Nutrition:
- Calories: 140 kcal
- Carbs: 0.6 g
- Protein: 25 g
- Fat: 2.6 g
- Sugar: 0.1 g
- Sodium: 73 mg
- Fiber: 0.1 g

Chapter 8.   Breakfast low fiber

42.   Spinach Frittata

Preparation Time: 10 minutes
Cooking Time: 30 minutes
Servings: 4
Ingredients:

- 2 teaspoons olive oil
- 1 cup red pepper, seeded and chopped
- 1 garlic clove, minced
- 3 cups spinach leaves, chopped
- 4 large eggs, beaten
- 1/2 teaspoon salt
- 1/4 cup Parmesan cheese, freshly grated

Directions:

1. Preheat the oven to 350ºF. In a non-stick oven pan, heat 1 teaspoon of olive oil over medium heat.
2. Cook red peppers and garlic until vegetables are soft (about 10 minutes). In a medium bowl, combine the eggs, spinach and salt; set aside.
3. Add remaining 1 teaspoon of olive oil into the pan with vegetables and add in the egg mixture.
4. Set the heat and cook for 15 minutes. Sprinkle Parmesan cheese over the mixture and broil for an additional 4 minutes.

Nutrition:
Calories: 106
Fat: 8 g
Carbs: 7 g
Fiber: 2 g
Protein: 3 g

43.   Banana and Pear Pita Pockets

Preparation Time: 10 minutes
Cooking Time: 0 minutes
Servings: 1
Ingredients:

- 1/2 small banana, peeled and sliced
- 1 round pita bread, made with refined white flour
- 1/2 small pear, peeled, seedless, cored, cooked and sliced
- 1/4 cup low-fat Cottage cheese

Directions:

1. Combine the banana, pear, and Cottage cheese in a small bowl. Slice the pita bread to make a pocket.
2. Fill it with the mixture.
3. Serve.

Nutrition:
Calories: 402
Fat: 2 g
Carbs: 87 g
Fiber: 11 g
Protein: 14 g

44.   Ripe Plantain Bran Muffins

Preparation Time: 10 minutes
Cooking Time: 20 minutes
Servings: 12
Ingredients:

- 1 ½ cup refined cereal
- 2/3 cup low-fat milk
- 4 large eggs, lightly beaten
- 1/4 cup canola oil
- 2 medium ripe plantains, mashed
- 1/2 cup brown sugar
- 1 cup refined white flour
- 2 teaspoons baking powder
- 1/2 teaspoon salt

Directions:

1. Preheat the oven to 400ºF. In a bowl, combine the bran cereal and milk; set aside.
2. Add eggs and oil; stir in brown sugar and mashed ripe plantain. In another bowl, combine salt, flour, and baking powder.
3. Dissolve the dry ingredients into the ripe plantain mixture, stir until combined.
4. Pour the batter evenly into paper-lined muffin tins; bake for 18 minutes or until golden brown and firm. Allow cooling before serving.

Nutrition:
Calories: 325
Fat: 19 g
Carbs: 37 g
Fiber: 2 g
Protein: 3 g

45.   Easy Breakfast Bran Muffins

Preparation Time: 10 minutes

Cooking Time: 20 minutes
Servings: 10
Ingredients:

- 2 cups refined cereal
- 1 cup boiling water
- 1/2 cup brown sugar
- 1/2 cup butter
- 2 eggs
- 1/2 quart buttermilk
- 2 ½ cups refined white flour
- 2 ½ teaspoons baking soda
- 1/2 teaspoon salt

Directions:

1. Preheat the oven to 400°F. Soak 1 cup of cereal in 1 cup of boiling water and set aside.
2. In a mixer, merge the brown sugar and butter until it is fully mixed. Add each egg separately and beat until fluffy. Then, stir in the buttermilk and the soaked cereal mixture.
3. In another bowl, combine salt, flour and baking soda. Add the flour mixture into the batter and ensure not to over mix.
4. Add in the remaining cup of cereal. Set the batter evenly into 10 greased or paper-lined muffin tins. Bake for 15-20 minutes. Allow cooling before serving.

Nutrition:
Calories: 440
Fat: 20 g
Carbs: 57 g
Fiber: 3 g
Protein: 9 g

46. Apple Oatmeal

Preparation Time: 10 minutes
Cooking Time: 1-2 minutes
Servings: 1
Ingredients:

- 1/2 cup instant oatmeal
- 3/4 cup milk or water
- 1/2 cup apples, peeled and cooked pureed
- 1 teaspoon brown sugar

Directions:

1. In a microwave-safe bowl, mix oats, milk or water and apples. Cook in a microwave on high.

2. Stir and cook for another 30 seconds. Sprinkle with brown sugar and add a splash of milk.

Nutrition:
Calories: 295
Fat: 7 g
Carbs: 47 g
Fiber: 5 g
Protein: 13 g

47. Breakfast Burrito Wrap

Preparation Time: 15 minutes
Cooking Time: 15 minutes
Servings: 1
Ingredients:

- 1 tablespoon extra-virgin olive oil
- 2 slices turkey bacon
- 1/4 cup green bell peppers, seeded and chopped
- 2 eggs, beaten
- 2 tablespoons milk
- 1/4 teaspoon salt
- 2 tablespoons low-fat Monterrey Jack cheese, grated
- 1 white tortilla

Directions:

1. In a small non-stick pan, warm olive oil on medium heat and cook the turkey for about 2 minutes until slightly crispy.
2. Attach bell peppers and continue to cook until warmed through. In a small bowl beat the eggs with milk and salt.
3. Gently, stir in your eggs until almost cooked through. Turn the heat down then add the cheese.
4. Cover and continue cooking until cheese has completely melted. Place the mixture on the tortilla and roll it into a burrito.

Nutrition:
Calories: 355
Fat: 2 g
Carbs: 14 g
Fiber: 4 g
Protein: 23 g

48. Zucchini Omelet

Preparation Time: 15 minutes
Cooking Time: 15 minutes
Servings: 4

Ingredients:

- 2 tablespoons extra-virgin olive oil
- 1 medium zucchini, seeded and cubed
- 1/2 medium tomato, seeded and chopped
- 4 large eggs
- 1/4 cup milk
- 1 teaspoon salt
- 4 whole-wheat English muffins

Directions:

1. In a large non-stick pan, warm olive oil over moderate heat. Add the zucchini and tomato.
2. Cook vegetables for 5-10 minutes or until they are soft.
3. In a separate bowl, merge the eggs, milk and salt.
4. Attach the egg mixture to the pan and stir to cook through. Set with white English muffins.

Nutrition:

Calories: 160

Fat: 10 g

Carbs: 14 g

Fiber: 2 g

Protein: 6 g

49. Coconut Chia Seed Pudding

Preparation Time: 15 minutes

Cooking Time: 0 minutes

Servings: 2

Ingredients:

- 6 tablespoons Chia seeds
- 2 cups coconut milk, unsweetened)
- Blueberries for topping

Directions:

1. Merge the chia seeds and milk; mix well. Refrigerate overnight.
2. Stir in the berries and serve.

Nutrition:

Calories: 223

Fat: 12 g

Carbs: 18 g

Fiber: 2 g

Protein: 10 g

50. Spiced Oatmeal

Preparation Time: 2 minutes

Cooking Time: 2 minutes

Servings: 2

Ingredients:

- 1/3 cup quick oats
- 1/4 teaspoon ground ginger
- 1/8 teaspoon ground cinnamon
- A dash of ground nutmeg
- A dash of ground clove
- 1 tablespoon almond butter
- 1 cup Water

Directions:

1. Combine the oats and water. Microwave for 45 seconds, then stir and cook for another 30-45 seconds.
2. Add in the spices and drizzle on the almond butter before serving.

Nutrition:

Calories: 467

Fat: 11 g

Carbs: 33 g

Fiber: 4 g

Protein: 6 g

51. Breakfast Cereal

Preparation Time: 5 minutes

Cooking Time: 5 minutes

Servings: 4

Ingredients:

- 3 cups cooked old fashioned oatmeal
- 3 cups cooked quinoa
- 4 cups bananas, peeled and chopped

Directions:

1. Combine the oatmeal and quinoa; mix well.
2. Evenly, divide into 4 bowls and top with the bananas before serving.

Nutrition:

Calories: 228

Fat: 3 g

Carbs: 43 g

Fiber: 6 g

Protein: 12 g

52. Sweet Potato Hash with Sausage and Spinach

Preparation Time: 5 minutes

Cooking Time: 15 minutes

Servings: 4

Ingredients:

- 4 small chopped sweet potatoes

- 2 apples, cored and chopped
- 1 garlic clove, minced
- 1 pound ground sausage
- 10 ounces chopped spinach
- Salt and pepper

Directions:
1. Brown the sausage until no pink remains. Add the remaining ingredients.
2. Cook until the spinach and apples are tender. Season to taste and serve hot.

Nutrition:
Calories: 544
Fat: 2 g
Carbs: 65 g
Fiber: 2 g
Protein: 11 g

53. Cajun Omelet

Preparation Time: 5 minutes
Cooking Time: 8 minutes
Servings: 2
Ingredients:

- 1/4 pound spicy sausage
- 1/3 cup sliced mushrooms
- 1/2 diced onion
- 4 large eggs
- 1/2 medium bell pepper, chopped
- 2 tablespoons water
- A pinch of cayenne pepper (optional)
- Sea salt and fresh pepper to taste
- 1 tbsp. Mustard

Directions:
1. Brown the sausage in a saucepan until cooked through. Add the mushrooms, onion and bell pepper. Cook for another 3-5 minutes, or until tender.
2. Meanwhile, whisk together the eggs, water, mustard and spices. Season with salt and pepper.
3. Top with your eggs over then reduce to low heat. Cook until the top is nearly set and then fold the omelet in half and cover.
4. Cook for another minute before serving hot.

Nutrition:
Calories: 467
Fat: 14 g
Carbs: 11 g
Fiber: 2 g

Protein:

54. Strawberry Cashew Chia Pudding

Preparation Time: 10 minutes
Cooking Time: 0 minutes
Servings: 2
Ingredients:

- 6 tablespoon chia seeds
- 2 cups cashew milk, unsweetened
- Strawberries, for topping

Directions:
1. Merge the chia seeds and milk; mix well. Refrigerate overnight.
2. Stir in the berries and serve.

Nutrition:
Calories: 223
Fat: 12 g
Carbs: 18 g
Fiber: 2 g
Protein: 10 g

55. Peanut Butter Banana Oatmeal

Preparation Time: 5 minutes
Cooking Time: 0 minutes
Servings: 1
Ingredients:

- 1/3 cup quick oats
- 1/4 teaspoon cinnamon (optional)
- 1/2 sliced banana
- 1 tablespoon peanut butter, unsweetened

Directions:
1. Merge all ingredients in a bowl with a lid. Refrigerate.

Nutrition:
Calories: 645
Fat: 32 g
Carbs: 65 g
Fiber: 5 g
Protein: 26 g

56. Overnight Peach Oatmeal

Preparation Time: 10 minutes
Cooking Time: 0 minutes
Servings: 2
Ingredients:

- 1/2 cup old fashioned oats

- 2/3 cup skim milk
- 1/2 cup plain Greek yogurt
- 1 tablespoon chia seeds
- 1/2 teaspoon Vanilla
- 1/2 cup peach, peeled and diced
- 1 medium banana, peeled and chopped

Directions:
1. Combine the oats, milk, yogurt, chia seeds and vanilla in a bowl with a lid.
2. Refrigerate for 12 hours.
3. Top with the fruits before serving.

Nutrition:
Calories: 282
Fat: 6 g
Carbs: 48 g
Fiber: 2 g
Protein: 10 g

57. Mediterranean Salmon and Potato Salad

Preparation Time: 15 minutes
Cooking Time: 18 minutes
Servings: 4
Ingredients:

- 1 pound red potatoes, peeled and cut into wedges
- 1/2 cup plus 2 tablespoons more extra-virgin olive oil
- 2 tablespoons balsamic vinegar
- 1 tablespoon fresh rosemary, minced
- 2 cups peas, cooked and drained
- 4 (4 ounces each) salmon fillets
- 2 tablespoons lemon juice
- 1/4 teaspoon salt
- 2 cups English cucumber, sliced and seedless

Directions:
1. In a saucepan, set water to a boil and cook potatoes until tender, about 10 minutes.
2. Drain and set potatoes back into the pan. To make the dressing, in a bowl, set together 1/2 cup of olive oil, vinegar and rosemary.
3. Combine potatoes and peas with the dressing. Set aside. In a separate medium pan, warm the remaining 2 tablespoons of olive oil over medium heat.
4. Attach salmon fillets and set with lemon juice and salt.

5. Cook on both sides or until fish flakes easily. To serve, place cucumber slices on a serving plate top with potato salad and fish fillets.

Nutrition:
Calories: 463
Fat: 4 g
Carbs: 75 g
Fiber: 18 g
Protein: 34 g

58. Pea Tuna Salad

Preparation Time: 15 minutes
Cooking Time: 0 minutes
Servings: 4
Ingredients:

- 3 pounds cooked peas
- 1/2 cup low-fat mayonnaise
- 1/3 cup tarragon vinegar
- 1 teaspoon honey Dijon mustard
- 2 small shallots, thinly sliced
- 2 (6 ounces) cans tuna fish, drained
- 2 small sprigs fresh tarragon, finely chopped

Directions:
1. In a large bowl, merge mayonnaise, vinegar and mustard. Add tuna fish, shallots and peas; toss to coat with dressing.
2. Secure and refrigerate for 1 hour before serving. Set with fresh tarragon and serve.

Nutrition:
Calories: 246
Fat: 13 g
Carbs: 11 g
Fiber: 1 g
Protein: 22 g

59. Vegetable Soup

Preparation Time: 15 minutes
Cooking Time: 1 hour 20 minutes
Servings: 2
Ingredients:

- 2 tablespoons extra-virgin olive oil
- 4 garlic cloves, finely chopped
- 2 celery stalks, finely sliced
- 2 carrots, finely sliced
- 6 cups water or chicken broth
- 1/4 teaspoon thyme
- 1/4 teaspoon rosemary
- 1 bay leaf

- 1 can (14 ounces) peas
- 1/2 teaspoon salt

Directions:
1. Warmth up the oil over medium heat in a soup pot. Add garlic, celery, and carrots and continue to cook for 5 minutes, stirring occasionally.
2. Add water or chicken broth, thyme, rosemary and bay leaf. Cook until it comes to a boil.
3. Set the heat and simmer gently for about 45-60 minutes. Add peas and season with salt.
4. Let soup cool slightly, remove the bay leaf and puree with a hand blender, until creamy.
5. Serve in warmed soup bowls.

Nutrition:
Calories: 242
Fat: 8 g
Carbs: 34 g
Fiber: 13 g
Protein: 12 g

60. Carrot and Turkey Soup

Preparation Time: 15 minutes
Cooking Time: 40 minutes
Servings: 4
Ingredients:

- 1/2 pound lean ground turkey
- 1/2 bag frozen carrot
- 1/4 cup green peas
- 1 can (32 ounces) chicken broth
- 2 medium tomatoes, seeded and roughly chopped
- 1 teaspoon garlic powder
- 1 teaspoon paprika
- 1 teaspoon oregano
- 1 bay leaf

Directions:
1. Over medium heat, set the ground turkey in a soup pot. Add peas, frozen carrot, paprika, tomatoes, garlic powder, bay leaf, oregano, and broth.
2. Set the pot to a boil, lower heat, cover, and simmer for 30 minutes.

Nutrition:
Calories: 436
Fat: 12 g
Carbs: 20 g
Fiber: 6 g

Protein: 59 g

61. Creamy Pumpkin Soup

Preparation Time: 15 minutes
Cooking Time: 1 hour 10 minutes
Servings: 4
Ingredients:

- 1 pumpkin, cut lengthwise, seeds removed and peeled
- 1 sweet potato, cut lengthwise and peeled
- 2 tablespoons olive oil
- 4 garlic cloves, unpeeled
- 4 cups vegetable stock
- 1/4 cup light cream
- Salt
- 1 tbsp. chopped Shallots

Directions:
1. Preheat the oven to 375°F. Cut all the sides of the pumpkin, shallots and sweet potato with oil.
2. Transfer your vegetables with the garlic to a roasting pan. Set to roast for about 40 minutes or until tender.
3. Let the vegetables cool for a time and scoop out the flesh of the sweet potato and pumpkin.
4. In a soup pot, place the flesh of roasted vegetables, shallots and peeled garlic. Add the broth and set to a boil.
5. Set the heat, and let it simmer, covered for 30 minutes, stirring occasionally. Let the soup cool.
6. Set the soup with a hand blender, until smooth. Add the cream.
7. Season to taste and simmer until warmed through, about 5 minutes. Serve in warm soup bowls.

Nutrition:
Calories: 332
Fat: 18 g
Carbs: 32 g
Fiber: 9 g
Protein: 12 g

62. Chicken Pea Soup

Preparation Time: 15 minutes
Cooking Time: 55 minutes
Servings: 4
Ingredients:

- 1 pound chicken breast, skinless, boneless and cubed
- 2 tablespoons olive oil
- 3 garlic cloves, minced
- 3 carrots, grated
- 1 bay leaf
- 1 teaspoon salt
- 1 teaspoon poultry seasoning
- 8 cups chicken broth
- 1/2 cup dried split peas, washed and drained
- 1 cup green peas

Directions:
1. Warmth up the olive oil over medium heat in a soup pot. Add the chicken and cook for 5 minutes, until lightly browned.
2. Attach the garlic, bay leaf, carrots, salt and seasoning. Cook until vegetables soften, stirring occasionally.
3. Pour the broth and split peas into the pot; bring to a boil. Set the heat, cover and simmer on low heat for 30-45 minutes.
4. Stir in green peas to the soup and heat for 5 minutes, stirring to combine all ingredients.

Nutrition:
Calories: 176
Fat: 5 g
Carbs: 18 g
Fiber: 6 g
Protein: 15 g

63. Coconut Pancakes

Preparation Time: 10 minutes
Cooking Time: 10 minutes
Servings: 2
Ingredients:
- 1/2 cup coconut milk, plus additional as needed
- 1/2 tablespoon maple syrup
- 1/4 cup coconut flour
- 1/2 teaspoon salt
- 2 eggs
- 1/2 tablespoon coconut oil or almond butter, plus additional for greasing the pan
- 1/2 teaspoon vanilla extract
- 1/2 teaspoon baking soda

Directions:
1. Using an electric mixer, combine the coconut milk, maple syrup, eggs, coconut oil, and vanilla in a medium mixing cup.
2. Combine the baking soda, coconut flour, and salt in a shallow mixing bowl.
3. Set the dry ingredients with the wet ingredients in a mixing bowl and beat until smooth and lump-free.
4. If the batter is too dense, add more liquid to thin it down to a typical pancake batter consistency.
5. Using coconut oil, lightly grease a big skillet or pan. Preheat the oven to medium-high.
6. Cook until golden brown on the rim for another 2 minutes.
7. Continue cooking the leftover batter while stacking the pancake on a tray.

Nutrition:
Calories: 193
Fat: 11 g
Carbs: 15 g
Sugar: 6 g
Fiber: 6 g
Protein: 9 g
Sodium: 737 mg

Chapter 9. Breakfast high fiber

64. Mango Ginger Smoothie

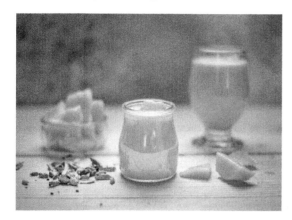

Preparation time: 5 minutes
Serving: 1
Ingredients:

- Red lentils – half cup, cooked cooled
- mango chunks – one cup, frozen
- Carrot juice – ¾ cup
- Fresh ginger – one tsp, chopped
- Honey – one tsp
- Ground cardamom – one pinch
- Ice cubes – three cubes

Directions:

1. Add all ingredients into the blender and blend on high, about two to three minutes.
2. Garnish with cardamom.

Nutrition:
Calories; 352kcal, Carbohydrates; 78.9g, Fats; 1.1g Proteins; 12.3g, fiber; 9.6g

65. Cherry Spinach Smoothie
Preparation time: 5 minutes
Serving: 1
Ingredients:

- Kefir – one cup, low-fat
- Frozen cherries – one cup
- Baby spinach leaves – half cup
- Avocado – ¼ cup, mashed
- Salted almond butter – one tbsp
- Ginger – ½-inch piece, peeled
- Chia seeds – one tsp

Directions:

1. Add all ingredients into the blender and blend on high, about two to three minutes.
2. Pour smoothie into the glass.
3. Garnish with chia seeds.

Nutrition:
Calories; 410kcal, Carbohydrates; 46.6g, Fats; 20.1g Proteins; 17.4g, fiber; 10.1g

66. Banana cacao smoothie

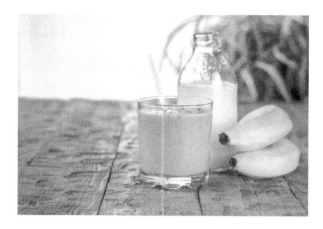

Preparation time: 5 minutes
Serving: 2
Ingredients:

- Frozen banana – two, sliced
- Cacao Bliss – ¼ cup
- Almond butter – ¼ cup
- Hemp hearts – 2 tbsp
- Non-dairy milk – 2 cups
- Ice – ½ cup

Directions:

1. Add all ingredients into the blender and blend on high, about two to three minutes.
2. Pour smoothie into the glass.

Nutrition:
Calories; 515kcal, Carbohydrates; 48g, Fats; 31g Proteins; 22g, fiber; 11g

67. Spinach and Egg Scramble with Raspberries

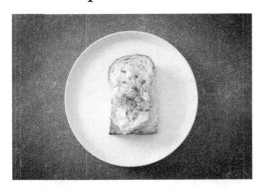

Preparation time: 10 minutes
Serving: 1
Ingredients:

- Canola oil – 1 tsp
- Baby spinach – 1 ½ cups
- Eggs – 2, beaten
- Kosher salt – one pinch
- ground pepper – one pinch
- Whole-grain bread – one slice, toasted
- Fresh raspberries – half cup

Directions:

1. Add oil into the skillet and heat it over medium-high flame.
2. Add spinach and cook for one to two minutes until wilted.
3. Transfer the spinach to the medium plate.
4. Clean the pan and place it over medium flame. Then, add eggs and cook for one to two minutes.
5. Add pepper, salt, and spinach and stir well.
6. Top with raspberries. Serve with toasted bread.

Nutrition:
Calories; 296kcal, Carbohydrates; 20.9g, Fats; 15.7g Proteins; 17.8g, fiber; 7g

68. Blackberry Smoothie

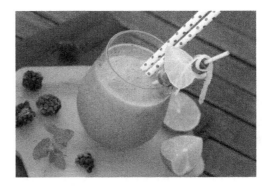

Preparation time: 5 minutes
Serving: 1
Ingredients:

- Fresh blackberries – one cup
- Banana – half
- Plain whole-milk Greek yogurt – half cup
- Honey – one tbsp
- Fresh lemon juice – 1 ½ tsp
- Fresh ginger – 1 tsp, chopped

Directions:

1. Add all ingredients into the blender and blend on high, about two to three minutes.
2. Pour smoothie into the glass.

Nutrition:
Calories; 316kcal, Carbohydrates; 53g, Fats; 7g Proteins; 15g, fiber; 10g

69. Veggie Frittata

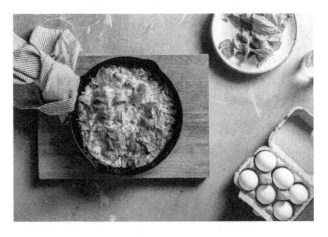

Preparation time: 5 minutes
Cooking time: 10 minutes
Serving: 1
Ingredients:

- Canola oil – one tbsp
- Scallions – two green and white parts separated, thinly sliced

- Mixed veggies – one cup carrots, broccoli, and cauliflower, chopped
- Salt – 1/8 tsp
- Eggs – 2, beaten
- Cheddar cheese – 2 tbsp, shredded
- Orange – 1, cut into wedges

Directions:
1. Add oil into a skillet and place it over medium-high flame.
2. Add salt, veggies, and whites scallions and cook for three to five minutes until browned. Add green scallions and stir well.
3. Pour eggs over the vegetables and sprinkle with cheese.
4. Cover with a foil and remove from the flame.
5. Let sit for four to five minutes.
6. Serve with orange wedges.

Nutrition:
Calories; 491kcal, Carbohydrates; 37g, Fats; 29g Proteins; 22g, fiber; 7g

70.   Chocolate Banana Protein Smoothie

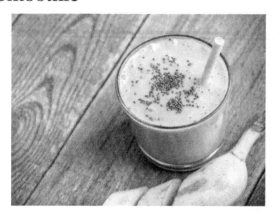

Preparation time: 5 minutes
Serving: 1
Ingredients:
- Banana – one, frozen
- Red lentils – half cup, cooked
- Milk – half cup, non-fat
- Unsweetened cocoa powder – 2 tsp
- Pure maple syrup – one tsp

Directions:
1. Mix the syrup, cocoa, milk, lentils, and banana into the blender and blend until smooth.
2. Serve!

Nutrition:
Calories; 310kcal, Carbohydrates; 63.8g, Fats; 1.8g Proteins; 15.3g, fiber; 8.5g

71.   Cocoa Almond French toast

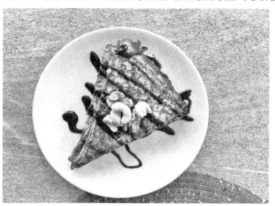

Preparation time: 10 minutes
Serving: 2
Ingredients:
- Unsweetened almond milk – ½ cup
- Egg – 1
- Ground cinnamon – ½ tsp
- Ground nutmeg – ½ tsp
- Almond – ¼ cup, chopped
- Non-stick cooking spray
- Whole wheat bread – four slices
- Chocolate syrup – 2 tbsp, sugar-free
- Raspberries – ¼ cup

Directions:
1. Add nutmeg, cinnamon, eggs, and almond milk into the dish and keep ½ tbsp of chopped almonds to garnish.
2. Place remaining chopped almonds in another bowl.
3. Let coat the griddle with a cooking spray.
4. Heat the griddle over medium flame.
5. Meanwhile, immerse each bread slice into the egg mixture.
6. Then, dip soaked bread in the almonds and coat on both sides.
7. Place coated bread slices onto the griddle and cook for four to six minutes until golden brown.
8. Cut bread in half, lengthwise. Place onto the two serving plates.
9. Drizzle with chocolate syrup.
10. Top with raspberries and chopped almonds.

Nutrition:

Calories; 250kcal, Carbohydrates; 28.6g, Fats; 11.7g Proteins; 15g, fiber; 7.9g

72.   Muesli with Raspberries

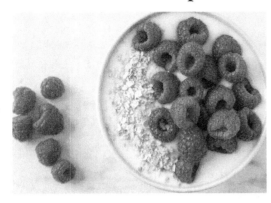

Preparation time: 5 minutes
Serving: 1
Ingredients:

- Muesli – 1/3 cup
- Raspberries – one cup
- Milk – ¾ cup, low-fat

Directions:
Place muesli into the bowl. Top with raspberries. Serve with warm or cold water.
Nutrition:
Calories; 288kcal, Carbohydrates; 51.8g, Fats; 6.6g Proteins; 13g, fiber; 13.3g

73.   Mocha Overnight Oats

Preparation time: 10 minutes
Chill time: 8 hours
Serving: 1
Ingredients:

- Rolled oats – half cup
- Milk – half cup, low fat
- Cooled coffee – ¼ cup
- Pure maple syrup – one tbsp
- Chia seeds – 1 ½ tsp
- Cocoa powder – 1 ½ tsp
- Walnuts – 1 tbsp, toasted, chopped
- Cacao nibs – one tsp

Directions:
Mix the cocoa powder, chia seeds, maple syrup, coffee, milk, and oats into the bowl. Cover with a lid and put it into the fridge overnight or for eight hours.

Top with cacao nibs and walnuts.
Nutrition:
Calories; 379kcal, Carbohydrates; 53g, Fats; 15.1g Proteins; 12.6g, fiber; 9.1g

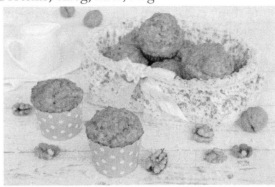

74.   Baked Banana-Nut Oatmeal Cups

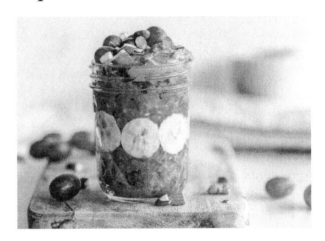

Preparation time: 10 minutes
Baking time: 25 minutes
Serving: 12
Ingredients:

- Rolled oats – three cups
- Low-fat milk – 1 ½ cups
- Bananas – two, mashed
- Brown sugar – 1/3 cup
- Eggs – two, beaten
- Baking powder – one tsp
- Ground cinnamon – one tsp
- Vanilla extract – one tsp
- Salt – half tsp

Pecans – half cup, chopped, toasted
Directions:

1. Preheat the oven to 375 degrees Fahrenheit.
2. Let coat the muffin tin with cooking spray.

3. Mix the salt, vanilla, cinnamon, baking powder, eggs, brown sugar, bananas, milk, and oats into the bowl.
4. Fold in the pecans. Place mixture into the muffin cups and bake for twenty-five minutes.
5. Let cool it for ten minutes.
6. Serve and enjoy!

Nutrition:
Calories; 176kcal, carbohydrates; 26.4g, protein; 5.2g, fat; 6.2g, fiber; 3.1g

75. Pineapple Green Smoothie

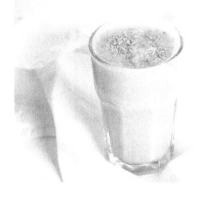

Preparation time: 5 minutes
Serving: 1
Ingredients:
- Unsweetened almond milk – half cup
- Plain Greek yogurt – 1/3 cup, non-fat
- Baby spinach – one cup
- Frozen banana slices – one cup
- Frozen pineapple chunks – half cup
- Chia seeds – one tbsp
- Pure maple syrup or honey – one to two tsp

Directions:
1. Add yogurt and almond milk into the blender and blend until smooth.
2. Then, add spinach, pineapple, bananas, honey or maple syrup, and chia into the blender and blend until smooth.

Serve and enjoy!

Nutrition:
Calories; 297kcal, carbohydrates; 54.3g, protein; 12.8g, fat; 5.7g, fiber; 9.8g

76. Pumpkin Bread

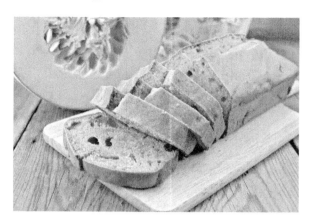

Preparation time: 10 minutes
Cooking time: 1 hour 15 minutes
Serving: 12
Ingredients:
- Water – five tbsp
- Flaxseed meal – two tbsp
- Unsweetened almond milk – ¾ cup
- Sugar – ¾ cup
- Canola oil – 1/3 cup
- Vanilla extract – one tsp
- Unseasoned pumpkin puree – 1 ½ cups
- White whole-wheat flour – two cups
- Baking powder – two tsp
- Pumpkin pie spice or cinnamon – one tsp
- Salt – half tsp
- Bittersweet chocolate chips – half cup

Directions:
1. Preheat the oven to 350 degrees Fahrenheit.
2. Let coat the loaf pan with cooking spray.
3. Mix the flaxseed meal and water into the bowl. Let sit for few minutes.
4. Whisk the flaxseed mixture, vanilla, oil, sugar, and almond milk into the bowl. Then, add pumpkin puree and stir well.
5. Whisk the salt, pumpkin pie spice, flour, and baking powder into the bowl. Add wet ingredients and stir well.
6. Add chocolate chips and stir well.
7. Transfer the batter to the pan. Bake for one hour and fifteen minutes.
8. Let cool it for one hour.
9. Serve and enjoy!

Nutrition:
Calories; 191kcal, carbohydrates; 30.5g, protein; 3.3g, fat; 7g, fiber; 3.3g

77. Banana-Bran Muffins

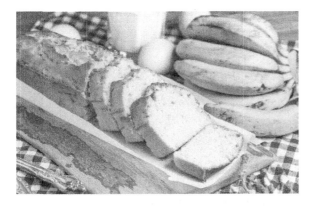

Preparation time: 10 minutes
Cooking time: 25 minutes
Serving: 12
Ingredients:

- Eggs – two
- Brown sugar – 2/3 cup
- Ripe bananas – one cup, mashed
- Buttermilk – one cup
- Unprocessed wheat bran – one cup
- Canola oil – ¼ cup
- Vanilla extract – one tsp
- Whole-wheat flour – one cup
- All-purpose flour – ¾ cup
- Baking powder – 1 ½ tsp
- Baking soda – half tsp
- Ground cinnamon – half tsp
- Salt – ¼ tsp
- Chocolate chips – half cup
- Walnuts – 1/3 cup, chopped

Directions:

- Preheat the oven to 400 degrees Fahrenheit.
- Let coat twelve muffin cups with cooking spray.
- Whisk the brown sugar and eggs into the bowl until smooth.
- Add vanilla, oil, wheat bran, buttermilk, and bananas and whisk it well.
- Whisk the salt, cinnamon, baking soda, baking powder, flour, all-purpose flour, and whole-wheat flour into the bowl.
- Make a well in the middle of the dry ingredients and then add wet ingredients and stir well.
- Add chocolate chips and stir well. Place batter into the muffin cups and sprinkle with

walnuts. Bake it for fifteen to twenty-five minutes until golden brown.

- Let cool it for five minutes.
- Serve and enjoy!

Nutrition:
Calories; 200kcal, carbohydrates; 34.1g, protein; 4.8g, fat; 7g, fiber; 3.9g

78. Banana Bread

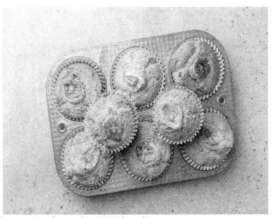

Preparation time: 15 minutes
Cooking time: 1 hour
Serving: 10
Ingredients:

- White whole-wheat flour – 1 ¾ cups
- Baking powder – 1 ½ tsp
- Ground cinnamon – one tsp
- Salt – half tsp
- Baking soda – ¼ tsp
- Sugar – ¾ cup
- Unsalted butter or coconut oil – ¼ cup, softened
- Eggs – two
- Ripe bananas – 1 ½ cups, mashed
- Buttermilk – ¼ cup
- Vanilla extract – one tsp
- Walnuts or chocolate chips – half cup, chopped

Directions:

1. Preheat the oven to 350 degrees Fahrenheit.
2. Let coat the loaf pan with cooking spray.
3. Whisk the baking soda, salt, cinnamon, flour, and baking powder into the bowl.
4. Add butter and sugar into the bowl and beat it well using an electric mixer over medium-high heat.

5. Add eggs and beat it well. Add flour mixture and beat on low speed and then fold in chocolate chips or walnuts.
6. Place batter into the pan. Bake for forty-five to fifty-five minutes.
7. Serve and enjoy!

Nutrition:
Calories; 221kcal, carbohydrates; 39.4g, protein; 4.7g, fat; 5.9g, fiber; 3.1g

79. Chocolate-Raspberry Oatmeal

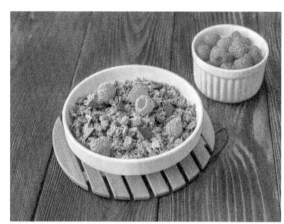

Preparation time: 10 minutes
Serving: 4
Ingredients:
- Regular rolled oats – 1 ½ cups
- Unsweetened cocoa powder – two tbsp
- Salt – ¼ tsp
- Unsweetened almond milk – three cups
- Fresh red raspberries – one cup
- Chocolate syrup – four tsp

Directions:
1. Add salt, cocoa powder, and oats into the saucepan. Add almond milk and stir well. Let boil it over medium flame. Lower the heat and simmer for five to seven minutes.
2. Remove from the flame. Let stand for two minutes.
3. Place oatmeal mixture into the serving bowls.
4. Top with ¼ cup of raspberries.
5. Drizzle with one tsp chocolate syrup.

Nutrition:
Calories; 157kcal, carbohydrates; 26.2g, protein; 5.4g, fat; 4.7g, fiber; 6.6g

80. Chai Chia Pudding

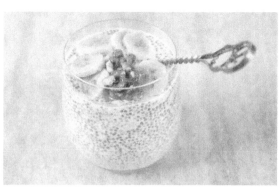

Preparation time: 10 minutes
Chill time: 8 hours
Serving: 1
Ingredients:
- Unsweetened almond milk – half cup
- Chia seeds – two tbsp
- Pure maple syrup – two tsp
- Vanilla extract – ¼ tsp
- Ground cinnamon – ¼ tsp
- Pinch of ground cardamom
- Pinch of ground cloves
- Banana – half cup, sliced
- Unsalted pistachios – one tbsp, chopped, roasted

Directions:
1. Add cloves, cardamom, cinnamon, vanilla, maple syrup, chia, and almond milk into the bowl and stir well.
2. Cover with a lid and place it into the refrigerator for eight hours.
3. When ready to serve, combine it well. Place half of the pudding into the glass and top with half of pistachios and bananas.
4. Then, add the remaining pudding and top with remaining pistachios and bananas.
5. Serve and enjoy!

Nutrition:
Calories; 264kcal, carbohydrates; 38.2g, protein; 6.3g, fat; 11.2g, fiber; 10.8g

81. Apple Cinnamon Oatmeal

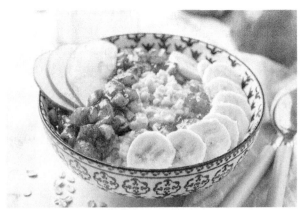

Preparation time: 5 minutes
Cooking time: 40 minutes
Serving: 4
Ingredients:

- Crisp apples – four
- Steel-cut oats – one cup
- Water – four cups
- Brown sugar – three tbsp
- Ground cinnamon – half tsp
- Salt – ¼ tsp
- Nonfat plain Greek yogurt – half cup

Directions:

1. Firstly, cut two apples with a box grater.
2. Add oats into the saucepan and cook over medium-high flame until toasted, for two minutes.
3. Then, add shredded apples and water and boil it.
4. Then, lower the heat and cook for ten minutes.
5. During this, chop two apples.
6. When oats have cooked, add salt, cinnamon, two tbsp brown sugar, chopped apples and stir well for fifteen to twenty minutes.
7. Place between four bowls.
8. Top with ¾ tsp brown sugar and two tbsp yogurt.

Nutrition:
Calories; 282kcal, carbohydrates; 59.1g, protein; 8g, fat; 2.7g, fiber; 6.3g

82. Apple Butter Bran Muffins

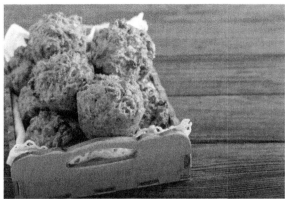

Preparation time: 5 minutes
Cooking time: 40 minutes
Serving: 12
Ingredients:

- Raisins – half cup
- Whole-wheat flour – ¾ cup
- All-purpose flour – ¾ cup
- Baking powder – 2 ½ tsp
- Salt – ¼ tsp
- Ground cinnamon – half tsp
- Unprocessed wheat bran – ¾ cup
- Egg – one, beaten
- Low-fat milk – half cup
- Spiced apple butter – half cup
- Brown sugar – half cup
- Canola oil – ¼ cup
- Molasses – three tbsp
- Apple – one cup, diced, peeled

Directions:

1. Preheat the oven to 375 degrees Fahrenheit.
2. Let coat twelve muffin cups with cooking spray.
3. Add raisins into the bowl and cover with hot water and keep it aside.
4. Whisk the cinnamon, salt, baking powder, flour, all-purpose flour, and whole-wheat flour into the bowl. Then, add bran and stir well.
5. Whisk the molasses, oil, brown sugar, apple butter, egg, and milk into the bowl. Make a well in the dry ingredients and place in the wet ingredients. Then, drain the raisins and add them to the bowl with diced apple. Stir well.
6. Place batter into the pan. Bake for eighteen to twenty-two minutes.
7. Let cool the pan for five minutes.

Serve and enjoy!
Nutrition:
Calories; 204kcal, carbohydrates; 37.6g, protein; 3.9g, fat; 5.7g, fiber; 3.7g

83. Pineapple Raspberry Parfaits

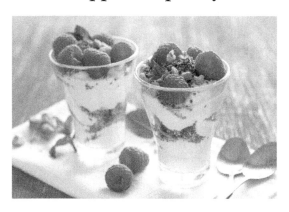

Preparation time: 5 minutes
Serving: 4
Ingredients:
- Nonfat peach yogurt – two cups
- Raspberries – half pint
- Pineapple chunks – 1 ½ cups

Directions:
Place pineapple, raspberries, and yogurt into the four glasses.
Serve and enjoy!
Nutrition:
Calories; 155kcal, carbohydrates; 33g, protein; 5.7g, fat; 0.5g, fiber; 2.9g

84. Berry Chia Pudding

Preparation time: 5 minutes
Chill time: 8 hours
Serving: 2
Ingredients:
- Blackberries, raspberries or diccd mango – 1 ¾ cups
- Unsweetened almond milk – one cup
- Chia seeds – ¼ cup
- Pure maple syrup – one tbsp
- Vanilla extract – ¾ tsp
- Whole-milk plain Greek yogurt – half cup
- Granola – ¼ cup

Directions:
Add milk and 1 ¼ cups fruit into the blender and blend until smooth.

Transfer it to the medium bowl. Add vanilla, syrup, and chia and combine well. Place it into the refrigerator for eight hours.
Place pudding into the two bowls. Layering each serving with two tbsp granola, ¼ cup yogurt, and remaining ¼ cup of fruit.
Serve!
Nutrition:
Calories; 343kcal, carbohydrates; 39.4g, protein; 13.8g, fat; 15.4g, fiber; 14.9g

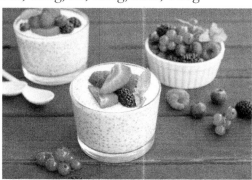

85. Spinach avocado smoothie

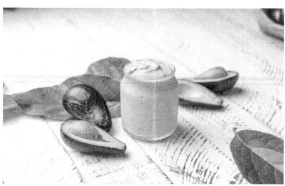

Preparation time: 5 minutes
Serving: 1
Ingredients:
- Nonfat plain yogurt – one cup
- Fresh spinach – one cup
- Banana – one, frozen
- Avocado – ¼
- Water – two tbsp
- Honey – one tsp

Directions:
1. Mix the honey, water, avocado, banana, spinach, and yogurt into the blender and blend until smooth.
2. Serve and enjoy!

Nutrition:
Calories; 357kcal, carbohydrates; 57.8g, protein; 17.7g, fat; 8.2g, fiber; 7.8g

86. Strawberry pineapple smoothie

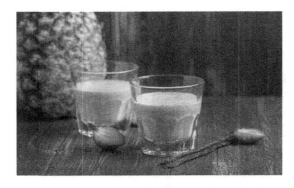

Preparation time: 5 minutes
Serving: 1
Ingredients:

- Frozen strawberries – one cup
- Fresh pineapple – one cup, chopped
- Unsweetened almond milk – ¾ cup, chilled
- Almond butter – one tbsp

Directions:

1. Mix the almond butter, almond milk, pineapple, and strawberries into the blender and process until smooth.
2. Add almond milk more if required.
3. Serve and enjoy!

Nutrition:
Calories; 255kcal, carbohydrates; 39g, protein; 5.6g, fat; 11.1g, fiber; 7.8g

87. Peach Blueberry Parfaits

Preparation time: 10 minutes
Serving: 2
Ingredients:

- Vanilla, Peach or blueberry fat-free yogurt – six ounce
- Sweetener multigrain clusters cereal – one cup
- Peach – one, pitted and sliced
- Fresh blueberries – half cup
- Ground cinnamon – ¼ tsp

Directions:

1. Add half of the yogurt into the two glasses.
2. Top with half of the cereal. Top with half of cinnamon, blueberries, and peaches. Place remaining blueberries, peaches, cereal, and yogurt.
3. Serve and enjoy!

Nutrition:
Calories; 166kcal, carbohydrates; 34g, protein; 11g, fat; 1g, fiber; 7g

88. Raspberry Yogurt Cereal Bowl

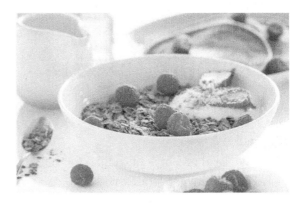

Preparation time: 5 minutes
Serving: 1
Ingredients:

- Nonfat plain yogurt – one cup
- Wheat cereal – half cup, shredded
- Fresh raspberries – ¼ cup
- Mini chocolate chips – two tsp
- Pumpkin seeds – one tsp
- Ground cinnamon – ¼ tsp

Directions:
Add yogurt into the bowl.
Top with cinnamon, pumpkin seeds, chocolate

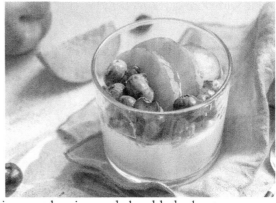

chips, raspberries, and shredded wheat.

Serve and enjoy!
Nutrition:
Calories; 290kcal, carbohydrates; 47.8g, protein; 18.4g, fat; 4.6g, fiber; 6g

89. Avocado toast

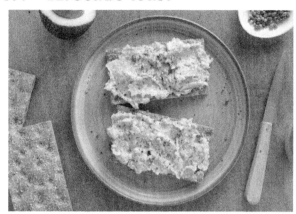

Preparation time: 10 minutes
Serving: 1
Ingredients:

- Mixed salad greens – one cup
- Red-wine vinegar – one tsp
- Extra-virgin olive oil – one tsp
- Pinch of salt
- Pinch of pepper
- Sprouted whole-wheat bread – two slices, toasted
- Plain hummus – ¼ cup
- Alfalfa sprouts – ¼ cup
- Avocado – ¼, sliced
- Unsalted sunflower seeds – two tsp

Directions:
Firstly, toss greens with pepper, salt, oil, and vinegar into the bowl.
Spread each slice of toast with two tbsp hummus and top with greens, sprouts, avocado, and spinach.
Sprinkle with sunflower seeds.
Serve and enjoy!
Nutrition:
Calories; 429kcal, carbohydrates; 46.4g, protein; 16.2g, fat; 21.9g, fiber; 15.1g

90. Loaded Pita Pockets

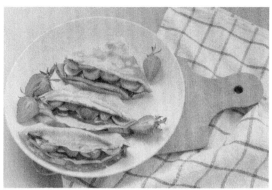

Preparation time: 5 minutes
Serving: 1
Ingredients:

- Whole wheat pita – one, halved
- Low-fat cottage cheese – half cup
- Walnut halves – four, chopped
- Banana – one, sliced

Directions:
Fill each pita with banana, walnuts, and cottage cheese.
Nutrition:
Calories; 307kcal, carbohydrates; 46g, protein; 21g, fat; 8.5g, fiber; 11g

91. Pear pancakes

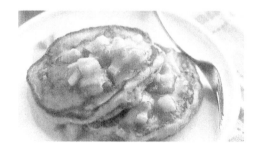

Preparation time: 10 minutes
Cooking time: 20 minutes
Servings: 4
Ingredients:

- One cup whole wheat flour
- ¼ teaspoon baking soda
- ¼ teaspoon baking powder
- One cup pears
- Two eggs
- One cup milk

Directions:

1.   In a bowl, combine all ingredients and mix well
2.   In a skillet, heat olive oil
3.   Pour ¼ of the batter and cook each pancake for 1-2 minutes per side
4.   When ready, remove from heat and serve
Nutrition: calories 277 fat 19g carbohydrates 56g protein 13.8g

92.   Almond pancakes
Preparation time: 10 minutes
Cooking time: 30 minutes
Servings: 4
Ingredients:
- One cup whole wheat flour
- ¼ teaspoon baking soda
- ¼ teaspoon baking powder
- One cup almonds
- Two eggs
- One cup milk

Directions:
1.   In a bowl, combine all ingredients and mix well
2.   In a skillet, heat olive oil
3.   Pour ¼ of the batter and cook each pancake for 1-2 minutes per side
4.   When ready, remove from heat and serve
Nutrition: calories 234g fat 20g carbohydrates 4.0g protein 10g

93.   Avocado pancakes
Preparation time: 10 minutes
Cooking time: 20 minutes
Servings: 4
Ingredients:
- One cup whole wheat flour
- ¼ teaspoon baking soda
- ¼ teaspoon baking powder
- Two eggs
- One cup milk
- 1cup mashed avocado

Directions:
1.   In a bowl, combine all ingredients and mix well
2.   In a skillet, heat olive oil
3.   Pour ¼ of the batter and cook each pancake for 1-2 minutes per side
4.   When ready, remove from heat and serve

Nutrition: calories 310 fat 18g carbohydrates 34g protein 7g

94.   Strawberry pancakes
Preparation time: 10 minutes
Cooking time: 20 minutes
Servings: 4
Ingredients:
- One cup whole wheat flour
- ¼ teaspoon baking soda
- ¼ teaspoon baking powder
- One cup strawberries
- Two eggs
- One cup milk

Directions:
1.   In a bowl, combine all ingredients and mix well
2.   In a skillet, heat olive oil
3.   Pour ¼ of the batter and cook each pancake for 1-2 minutes per side
4.   When ready, remove from heat and serve
Nutrition: calories 102 fat 4.7g carbohydrates 12g protein 3g

95.   Carambola pancakes
Preparation time: 10 minutes
Cooking time: 30 minutes
Servings: 4
Ingredients:
- One cup whole wheat flour
- ¼ teaspoon baking soda
- ¼ teaspoon baking powder
- Two eggs
- One cup milk
- One cup carambola

Directions:
1.   In a bowl, combine all ingredients and mix well
2.   In a skillet, heat olive oil
3.   Pour ¼ of the batter and cook each pancake for 1-2 minutes per side
4.   When ready, remove from heat and serve
Nutrition: calories 774 fat 35g carbohydrates 108g protein 5.89g

96.   Ginger muffins
Preparation time: 10 minutes
Cooking time: 20 minutes
Servings: 8-12

Ingredients:

- Two eggs
- One tablespoon olive oil
- One cup milk
- Two cups whole wheat flour
- One teaspoon baking soda
- ¼ teaspoon baking soda
- One teaspoon ginger
- One teaspoon cinnamon
- ¼ cup molasses

Directions:

1. In a bowl, combine all dry ingredients
2. In another bowl, combine all dry ingredients
3. Combine wet and dry ingredients
4. Fold in ginger and mix well
5. Pour mixture into 8-12 prepared muffin cups, fill 2/3 of the cups
6. Bake for 18-20 minutes at 375 f
7. When ready, remove from the oven and serve

Nutrition: calories 18707 fat 6.4g carbohydrates 29.0g protein 6.1g

97.   Carrot muffins

Preparation time: 10 minutes
Cooking time: 20 minutes
Servings: 8-12
Ingredients:

- Two eggs
- One tablespoon olive oil
- One cup milk
- Two cups whole wheat flour
- One teaspoon baking soda
- ¼ teaspoon baking soda
- One teaspoon cinnamon
- One cup carrots

Directions:

1. In a bowl, combine all dry ingredients
2. In another bowl, combine all dry ingredients
3. Combine wet and dry ingredients
4. Pour mixture into 8-12 prepared muffin cups, fill 2/3 of the cups
5. Bake for 18-20 minutes at 375 f
6. When ready, remove from the oven and serve

Nutrition: calories 342 fat 12.89g carbohydrates 50.3g protein 6.85

98.   Blueberry muffins

Preparation time: 10 minutes
Cooking time: 20 minutes
Servings: 8-12 minutes
Ingredients:

- Two eggs
- One tablespoon olive oil
- One cup milk
- Two cups whole wheat flour
- One teaspoon baking soda
- ¼ teaspoon baking soda
- One teaspoon cinnamon
- One cup blueberries

Directions:

1. In a bowl, combine all dry ingredients
2. In another bowl, combine all dry ingredients
3. Combine wet and dry ingredients
4. Fold in blueberries and mix well
5. Pour mixture into 8-12 prepared muffin cups, fill 2/3 of the cups
6. Bake for 18-20 minutes at 375 f, when ready remove and serve

Nutrition: calories 467 fat 13g carbohydrates 68g protein 6g

99.   Coconut muffins

Preparation time: 10 minutes
Cooking time: 20 minutes
Servings: 8-12
Ingredients:

- Two eggs
- One tablespoon olive oil
- One cup milk
- Two cups whole wheat flour
- One teaspoon baking soda
- ¼ teaspoon baking soda
- One teaspoon cinnamon
- One cup coconut flakes

Directions:

1. In a bowl, combine all dry ingredients
2. In another bowl, combine all dry ingredients
3. Combine wet and dry ingredients
4. Fold in blueberries and mix well
5. Pour mixture into 8-12 prepared muffin cups, fill 2/3 of the cups
6. Bake for 18-20 minutes at 375 f, when ready remove and serve

Nutrition: calories 130 fat 12g carbohydrates 0g protein 1g

100. Raisin muffin
Preparation time: 10 minutes
Cooking time: 20minutes
Servings: 8-12
Ingredients:

- Two eggs
- One tablespoon olive oil
- One cup milk
- Two cups whole wheat flour
- One teaspoon baking soda
- ¼ teaspoon baking soda
- One teaspoon cinnamon
- One cup raisins

Directions:
1. In a bowl, combine all dry ingredients
2. In another bowl, combine all dry ingredients
3. Combine wet and dry ingredients
4. Fold in blueberries and mix well
5. Pour mixture into 8-12 prepared muffin cups, fill 2/3 of the cups
6. Bake for 18-20 minutes at 375 f, when ready remove and serve
Nutrition: calories 502 fat 17g carbohydrates 79g protein 3.9g

101. Parmesan omelete
Preparation time: 5 minutes
Cooking time: 10 minutes
Servings: 1
Ingredients:

- Two eggs
- ¼ teaspoon salt
- ¼ teaspoon black pepper
- One tablespoon olive oil
- ¼ cup parmesan cheese
- ¼ teaspoon basil

Directions:
1. In a bowl, combine all ingredients and mix well
2. In a skillet, heat olive oil and pour the egg mixture
3. Cook for 1-2 minutes per side
4. When ready, remove the omelet from the skillet and serve
Nutrition: calories 291 fat 21.7g carbohydrates 1.9g protein 22g

102. Asparagus omelet
Preparation time: 5 minutes
Cooking time: 10 minutes
Servings: 1
Ingredients:

- Two eggs
- ¼ teaspoon salt
- ¼ teaspoon black pepper
- One tablespoon olive oil
- ¼ cup cheese
- ¼ teaspoon basil
- One cup asparagus

Directions:
1. In a bowl, combine all ingredients and mix well
2. In a skillet, heat olive oil and pour the egg mixture
3. Cook for 1-2 minutes per side
4. When ready, remove the omelet from the skillet and serve
Nutrition: calories 102.5 fat 5.1g carbohydrates 3.3g protein 10.3g

103. Onion omelet

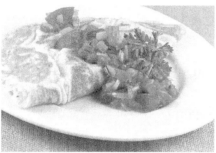

Preparation time: 5 minutes
Cooking time: 10 minutes
Servings: 1
Ingredients:

- Two eggs
- ¼ teaspoon salt
- ¼ teaspoon black pepper
- One tablespoon olive oil
- ¼ cup cheese
- ¼ teaspoon basil
- One cup red onion

Directions:
1. In a bowl, combine all ingredients and mix well
2. In a skillet, heat olive oil and pour the egg mixture
3. Cook for 1-2 minutes per side
4. When ready, remove the omelet from the skillet and serve
Nutrition: calories 200 fat 15g carbohydrates 4.6 protein 7.2g

104. Olive omelete
Preparation time: 5 minutes
Cooking time: 10 minutes
Servings: 1
Ingredients:

- Two eggs
- ¼ teaspoon salt
- ¼ teaspoon black pepper
- One tablespoon olive oil
- ¼ cup cheese
- ¼ teaspoon basil
- ½ cup olives

Directions:
1. In a bowl, combine all ingredients and mix well

2. In a skillet, heat olive oil and pour the egg mixture
3. Cook for 1-2 minutes per side
4. When ready, remove the omelet from the skillet and serve
Nutrition: calories 183 fat 13.8 carbohydrates 4g protein 15g

105. Tomato omelet

Preparation time: 5 minutes
Cooking time: 10 minutes
Servings: 1
Ingredients:

- Two eggs
- ¼ teaspoon salt
- ¼ teaspoon black pepper
- One tablespoon olive oil
- ¼ cup cheese
- ¼ teaspoon basil
- One cup tomatoes

Directions:
1. In a bowl, combine all ingredients and mix well
2. In a skillet, heat olive oil and pour the egg mixture
3. Cook for 1-2 minutes per side
4. When ready, remove the omelet from the skillet and serve
Nutrition: calories 456 fat 33g carbohydrates 13g protein 18.4g

106. Morning bagel
Preparation time: 5 minutes
Cooking time: 5 minutes
Servings: 1
Ingredients:

- One bagel
- One tablespoon cream cheese
- 2-3 tomato slices
- 1-2 onion slices

Directions:
1. Slice bagel and spread cream cheese over half
2. Place tomato slices and onion over one half
3. Top with the other half and serve
Nutrition: calories 289 fat 2g carbohydrates 56g protein 11g

107. Oatmeal custard

Preparation time: 5 minutes
Cooking time: 5 minutes
Servings: 1
Ingredients:

- ½ cup oatmeal
- ¼ cup coconut milk
- ¼ teaspoon cinnamon
- ¼ pear

Directions:
1. In a mug, combine oats, milk, pear, and almonds
2. Microwave for 3-4 minutes
3. When ready, remove and serve

Nutrition: calories 140 fat 2.5g carbohydrates 28g protein 5g

108. Scrambled eggs

Preparation time: 10 minutes
Cooking time: 10 minutes
Servings: 1
Ingredients:

- Six eggs
- ½ cup low-fat milk
- ¼ teaspoon salt
- ¼ teaspoon pepper
- One tablespoon butter
- ½ cup cream cheese
- ½ cup parmesan cheese

Directions:
1. In a bowl, whisk together eggs, salt, milk, and pepper
2. In a skillet, pour the egg mixture and sprinkle cream cheese and cook for 2-3 minutes per side
3. Remove and serve with parmesan cheese

Nutrition: calories 91 fat 6.7 carbohydrates 1.6g protein 10g

109. French toast

Preparation time: 5minutes
Cooking time: 10 minutes
Servings: 2
Ingredients:

- Two bread slices
- One teaspoon unsalted butter
- One egg
- ½ almond milk

Directions:
1. In a bowl, combine all ingredients for the dipping
2. Place the bread slices in the bowl and let the bread soak for 3-4 minutes
3. Fry in a skillet for 2-3 minutes per side
4. When ready, remove from the skillet and serve

Nutrition: calories 229 fat 11g carbohydrates 25g protein 8g

110. Simple pizza recipe

Preparation time: 10minutes
Cooking time: 15 minutes
Servings: 6-8
Ingredients:

- One pizza crust
- ½ cup tomato sauce
- ¼ black pepper
- One cup pepperoni slices
- One cup mozzarella cheese
- One cup olives

Directions:
1. Spread tomato sauce on the pizza crust
2. Place all the toppings on the pizza crust
3. Bake the pizza at 425 f for 12-15 minutes
4. When ready, remove pizza from the oven and serve

Nutrition: calories 266 fat 10g carbohydrates 33g protein 11g

111. Zucchini pizza

Preparation time: 10 minutes
Cooking time: 15 minutes
Servings: 6-8
Ingredients:

- One pizza crust
- ½ cup tomato sauce
- ¼ black pepper
- One cup zucchini slices
- One cup mozzarella cheese
- One cup olives

Directions:
1. Spread tomato sauce on the pizza crust
2. Place all the toppings on the pizza crust
3. Bake the pizza at 425 f for 12-15 minutes
4. When ready, remove pizza from the oven and serve

Nutrition: calories 121 fat 13g carbohydrates 31g protein 11g

112. Leeks fritatta

Preparation time: 10 minutes
Cooking time: 20 minutes
Servings: 2
Ingredients:

- ½ lb. Leek
- One tablespoon olive oil
- ½ red onion
- ¼ teaspoon salt
- Two eggs
- 2 oz. Cheddar cheese
- One garlic clove
- ¼ teaspoon dill

Directions:
1.   In a bowl, whisk eggs with salt and cheese
2.   In a frying pan, heat olive oil and pour egg mixture
3.   Add remaining ingredients and mix well
4.   Serve when ready
Nutrition: calories 225 fat 14.3g carbohydrates 9.7g protein 15g

113. Mushroom fritatta

Preparation time: 10 minutes
Cooking time: 20 minutes
Servings: 2
Ingredients:

- ½ lb. Mushrooms
- One tablespoon olive oil
- ½ red onion
- ¼ teaspoon salt
- Two eggs
- 2 oz. Cheddar cheese
- One garlic clove
- ¼ teaspoon dill

Directions:
1.   In a bowl, whisk eggs with salt and cheese
2.   In a frying pan, heat olive oil and pour egg mixture
3.   Add remaining ingredients and mix well
4.   Serve when ready
Nutrition: calories 456 fat g carbohydrates g protein g

114. Peas fritatta

Preparation time: 10 minutes
Cooking time: 20 minutes
Servings: 2
Ingredients:

- One cup peas
- One tablespoon olive oil
- ½ red onion
- ¼ teaspoon salt
- Two eggs
- 2 oz. Cheddar cheese
- One garlic clove
- ¼ teaspoon dill

Directions:
1.   In a bowl, whisk eggs with salt and cheese
2.   In a frying pan, heat olive oil and pour egg mixture
3.   Add remaining ingredients and mix well
4.   Serve when ready
Nutrition: calories 110 fat 6.2g carbohydrates 4.9g protein 8.5g

Chapter 10. Lunch clear liquid

115. Banana oat shake

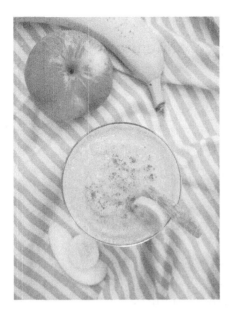

Preparation Time: 20 minutes
Cooking Time: 0 minutes
Total time: 20 minutes
Servings: 2

Ingredients:
- 1/2 cup cooked oatmeal, chilled
- 2/3 cup skim milk
- 2 tablespoons brown sugar
- 1 tablespoon wheat germ
- 1 1/2 teaspoons vanilla extract
- 1/2 frozen banana, cut into chunks

Directions:
1.   Blend the oatmeal for a few minutes in a blender.
2.   Mix in the milk, brown sugar, wheat germ, vanilla extract, and 1/2 banana. Blend until the mixture is thick and smooth.
3.   If desired, serve with ice.
Nutrition facts: calories: 173 | carbohydrates: 33 g | protein: 6 g | fat: 1 g | cholesterol: 150 mg

116. Banana-apple smoothie
Preparation Time: 15 minutes
Cooking Time: 0 minutes
Total time: 15 minutes
Servings: 1

Ingredients:

- 1/2 banana, peeled & cut into chunks
- 1/2 cup plain yogurt
- 1/2 cup unsweetened applesauce
- 1/4 cup skim milk
- 1 tablespoon honey
- 2 tablespoons oat bran

Directions:
1.   In a blender, combine the banana, yogurt, applesauce, milk, and honey.
2.   Blend until completely smooth.
3.   Blend in the oat bran until it is thickened.
Nutrition facts: calories: 292 | carbohydrates: 61 g | protein: 9 g | fat: 17 g | cholesterol: 103 mg

117. Berrylicious smoothie
Preparation Time: 20 minutes
Cooking Time: 0 minutes
Total time: 20 minutes
Servings: 2

Ingredients:
- 1/4 cup cranberry juice cocktail
- 2/3 cup silken tofu, firm
- 1/2 cup raspberries, frozen, unsweetened
- 1/2 cup blueberries, frozen, unsweetened
- 1 teaspoon vanilla extract
- 1/2 teaspoon powdered lemonade, such as country time

Directions:
1.   Fill a blender halfway with juice.
2.   Combine the remaining ingredients.
3.   Blend until completely smooth.
4.   Serve right away and enjoy!
Nutrition facts: calories: 115 | carbohydrates: 18 g | protein: 6 g | fat: 3 g | cholesterol: 223 mg

118. Buttermilk herb ranch dressing
Preparation Time: 10 minutes
Cooking Time: 0 minutes
Total time: 10 minutes
Servings: 2

Ingredients:
- 1/2 cup mayonnaise
- 1/2 cup milk
- 2 tablespoons vinegar

- 1 tablespoon fresh chives, chopped
- 1 tablespoon dill
- 1 tablespoon oregano leaves, chopped
- 1/4 teaspoon garlic powder

Directions:

1. In a medium mixing dish, combine mayonnaise, milk, and vinegar.
2. Then, with 1/4 teaspoon garlic powder, add fresh chives, dill, and oregano leaves.
3. Combine everything.
4. Allow at least one hour for flavors to emerge.
5. Before serving, thoroughly mix the dressing.

Nutrition facts: calories: 83 | carbohydrates: 1 g | protein: 1 g | fat: 6 g | cholesterol: 64 mg
Nutrition facts

119. Citrus relish

Preparation Time: 10 minutes
Cooking Time: 2 minutes
Total time: 12 minutes
Servings: 8

Ingredients:

- 2 pounds small lemons, limes, kumquats or oranges
- 1-quart white vinegar
- 1/4 cup mustard
- Glass jars
- 2-4 tablespoons sugar

Directions:

Pickled fruit

1. At the stem end of each fruit, make a cross. Quarter the oranges if using.
2. Fill glass jars halfway with vinegar.
3. To each jar, add 2 tablespoons of mustard. Put on the lids.
4. Allow it to sit at room temperature for about a month before preparing the relish listed below and serving.

Citrus relish

1. In a small frying pan, combine the fruit and sugar; add additional sugar to taste.
2. 5-10 minutes, shake the pan often over medium heat until the mixture boils and the fruit turns glossy and transparent.
3. Serve hot or cold.

4. The vinegar left over from the pickled fruit can be used to make salad dressing or to marinade chicken or seafood.

Nutrition facts: calories: 26 | carbohydrates: 7 g | protein: 0 g | fat: 0 g | cholesterol: 37 mg

120. Chickpea pancakes recipe

Preparation Time: 10 minutes
Cooking Time: 15 minutes
Total time: 25 minutes
Servings: 23

Ingredients:

- 1 cup (120g) chickpea flour
- 1 1/2 cups 375ml water
- 2 tablespoon olive oil *see note 1
- 1 carrot, finely grated
- 1/4 red capsicum, finely chopped
- 1 spring onion, finely chopped
- 1/4 tablespoon turmeric
- 1/4 tablespoon cumin
- 2 tablespoon chopped coriander (cilantro)
- 1/4 tablespoon salt

Directions:

7. In a mixing basin, combine the chickpea flour and water, constantly stirring to create a smooth, lump-free batter. Set aside.
8. Heat 1/2 tablespoon of the oil in a frying pan over medium-high heat. Combine the carrot, onion, turmeric, and cumin in a mixing bowl. Reduce the heat to medium-low and continue to simmer until the vegetables are softened (around 4-5 mins)
9. Combine the carrot mixture, chopped coriander, and salt in the chickpea batter (if using). Stir until everything is well mixed.
10. over medium-high heat, heat a nonstick frying pan. When the pan is heated, pour in the olive oil (or alternatively, use spray oil). Place a tablespoon of batter in the pan and spread it out with the back of your spoon (to make them thinner). To fill the pan, repeat the process. (*please see note 3)
11. cook each side for about 2 minutes (this will vary depending on the pan, heat, and how thin your pancake is). Look for bubbles to develop (as seen above), and your pancakes should be able to be easily flipped.

12. remove the pancakes from the pan and continue with the rest of the batter.

Nutrition facts: calories: 32 | carbohydrates: 3 g | protein: 1 g | fat: 1 g | cholesterol: 27 mg

121. Red wine sangria recipe
Preparation Time: 15 minutes
Cooking Time: 15 minutes
Total time: 30 minutes
Servings: 8

Ingredients:
- 750 ml rioja wine
- 3/4 cup solerno blood orange liqueur
- 3/4 cup leblon cachaca brazilian rum
- 1 1/2 cup orange juice
- 3/4 cup cherry juice
- 3/4 cup simple syrup sugar syrup
- 1/2 cup fresh lime juice
- 1 1/2 cups watermelon balls
- 1 cup raspberries
- 1 cup blackberries
- 2 mandarin oranges sliced
- 1 lime sliced
- 1 bunch basil leaves

Directions:
1. Stir together all of the liquid ingredients in a large pitcher. Then, to the pitcher, add the fresh fruit.
2. Refrigerate for at least 2 hours, covered. Pour into glasses and garnish with fresh basil leaves when ready to serve.

Nutrition facts: calories: 360 | carbohydrates: 51 g | protein: 1 g | fat: 1 g | cholesterol: 423 mg

122. Salty dog cocktail recipe
Preparation Time: 3 minutes
Cooking Time: 0 minutes
Total time: 3 minutes
Servings: 2

Ingredients:
- Four oz ruby red grapefruit juice
- Two oz vodka
- One ounce club soda or sparkling grapefruit-flavored water
- 1-2 teaspoons simple syrup
- Ice

- For garnish: kosher salt or fleur de sel agave syrup, grapefruit wedges

Directions:
1. Set out two tiny shallow plates for the salt rim. In one plate, spread salt, and in the other, spread a thin layer of agave syrup (or just syrup). Dip the edge of a highball glass in the syrup before dipping it in the salt.
2. Fill the glass three-quarters full of ice for each cocktail. Combine the grapefruit juice, vodka, club soda, and 1 teaspoon simple syrup in a mixing bowl.
3. Use a cocktail swizzle stick to stir. If desired, add a bit extra simple syrup to taste. Serve with a fresh grapefruit slice on the rim.
Notes: add a sprinkle of cayenne to the salt before dipping for a fiery salty dog.

Nutrition facts: calories: 202 | carbohydrates: 18 g | protein: 1 g | fat: 11 g | cholesterol: 26 mg

123. Simple syrup
Preparation Time: 2 minutes
Cooking Time: 3 minutes
Total time: 5 minutes
Servings: 8

Ingredients:
- 1 cup water
- 1 cup granulated sugar or turbinado, demerara

Directions:
1. Heat a small saucepot on high. Fill the saucepan halfway with water and sugar.
2. Bring to a boil, stirring constantly. Once boiling, remove from heat and stir. (if using herbs for infusion, add them to the simple boiling syrup.)
3. Allow cooling to room temperature before storing in an airtight container.
Nutrition facts: calories: 97 | carbohydrates: 25 g | protein: 2 g | fat: 12 g | cholesterol: 44 mg

124. Rose sangria recipe
Preparation Time: 15 minutes
Cooking Time: 0 minutes
Total time: 15 minutes
Servings: 8

Ingredients:
- 750 ml french rosé wine (1 bottle)

- 1 cup pink grapefruit juice
- 3/4 cup bourbon
- 1/2 cup honey
- 1/4 cup chambord (raspberry liqueur)
- 2 cups watermelon balls
- 1 1/2 cups fresh sliced strawberries
- 6 oz fresh raspberries

Directions:

1. Scoop 2 cups of watermelon balls from a big piece of fresh watermelon using a melon baller. Strawberries, sliced

2. In a large pitcher, combine the rosé wine, grapefruit juice, whiskey, honey, and chambord. Stir the honey into the mixture until it melts. (if your honey is particularly thick, reheat it first to thin it up before adding to the recipe.) After that, toss in the watermelon balls and strawberries. Refrigerate for at least 2 hours, covered.

3. Stir and taste for sweetness after at least two hours. If you want your sangria sweeter, add a bit, extra honey. If the sangria is too powerful, serve it over ice. When ready to serve, mix in the fresh raspberries and divide among glasses.

Nutrition facts: calories: 209 | carbohydrates: 26 g | protein: 0 g | fat: 0 g | cholesterol: 180 mg

125. Champagne holiday punch recipe

Preparation Time: 2 minutes
Cooking Time: 5 minutes
Total time: 7 minutes
Servings: 16

Ingredients:

- 750 ml of champagne (1 bottle)
- 24 oz ginger beer (2 bottles)
- Three cups of cranberry juice cocktail (or juice blend)
- Two cups of ruby red grapefruit juice
- One cup of spiced rum, optional
- Possible garnishes: fresh cranberries, grapefruit slices, cinnamon sticks

Directions:

1. All ingredients should be chilled. When ready to serve, combine all of the ingredients in a punch bowl.

2. Serve with cranberries, grapefruit slices, and cinnamon sticks as garnish.

Nutrition facts: calories: 107 | carbohydrates: 13 g | protein: 0 g | fat: 0 g | cholesterol: 0 mg

126. White sangria

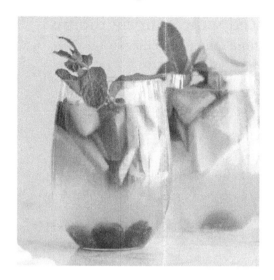

Preparation Time: 10 minutes
Cooking Time: 10 minutes
Total time: 20 minutes
Servings: 10

Ingredients:

- 750 ml moscato wine riesling is my second choice
- 1 1/2 cups orange-pineapple juice
- 1 cup domaine de canton ginger liqueur
- 1/2 cup midori melon liqueur
- 1 cup cantaloupe balls
- 1 cup sliced strawberries
- 2 mandarin oranges sliced
- 1 lime sliced
- 1-liter club soda chilled

Directions:

1. In a large pitcher, combine the wine, juice, and liqueurs. Refrigerate for at least 1 hour after adding the fruit.

2. Pour into glasses 2/3 full (scoop in some fruit) and top with club soda when ready to serve. Serve chilled.

Nutrition facts: calories: 218 | carbohydrates: 27 g | protein: 1 g | fat: 1 g | cholesterol: 18 mg

127. Raspberry mojitos with basil

Preparation Time: 10 minutes
Cooking Time: 10 minutes
Total time: 20 minutes

Servings: 8

Ingredients:

- One cup simple syrup 3/4 cup sugar + 3/4 cup water, heated to dissolve
- 1/2 cup torn basil leaves
- One cup fresh key lime juice use regular limes for slightly less acidity
- One cup white rum
- 1/4 cup chambord raspberry liquor
- 1-liter club soda
- Ice
- Fresh raspberries and lime slices to garnish

Directions:

1. In a large pitcher, combine the simple cooled syrup and the torn basil leaves. Muddle the basil leaves with a big spoon/ladle to unleash their flavor—beat them up quite hard.
2. Combine the lime juice, rum, and chambord in a mixing glass. Stir. Stir in the club soda and top with ice if the pitcher permits.
3. Garnish each glass with fresh berries and lime slices to serve. Serve cold with or without ice.

Nutrition facts: calories: 283 | carbohydrates: 36 g | protein: 1 g | fat: 1 g | cholesterol: 53 mg

128. Margarita recipe

Preparation Time: 10 minutes
Cooking Time: 10 minutes
Total time: 20 minutes
Servings: 10

Ingredients:

- 18 oz tequila blanco
- 18 oz fresh-squeezed lime juice (could be fresh bottled lime juice from the refrigerated section, but not the concentrated kind. Fresh)
- Nine oz la belle or grand marnier
- Eight oz simple syrup + a little extra for glass rims
- Three oz orange juice
- Three oz triple sec
- Coarse or flake sea salt for glass rims
- Sliced lime and orange for garnish

Directions:

1. If you don't have any on hand, start by preparing some simple syrup. 7 oz sugar and 7 oz water microwave until the sugar is completely dissolved. You should have around 9-10 oz left over for rimming the glasses.
2. Combine all of the margarita ingredients in a big pitcher. Chill after thoroughly stirring.
3. Pour the simple leftover syrup into a shallow dish when ready to serve. In a second shallow dish, add sea salt (or flake salt). Then, dip the rims of the glasses in simple syrup, followed by salt.
4. If preferred, add ice to the glasses, and fill a shaker halfway with ice. Shake the margarita mix for 10-15 seconds in a shaker. Pour into serving glasses. Serve the cups garnished with cut limes or oranges. Ole'!

Nutrition facts: calories: 300 | carbohydrates: 32 g | protein: 0 g | fat: 0 g | cholesterol: 29 mg

129. Grapefruit basil sorbet

Preparation Time: 35 minutes
Cooking Time: 20 minutes
Total time: 55 minutes
Servings: 6

Ingredients:

- Four large ruby red grapefruits, juiced
- Two cups of water
- 1 3/4 cups of organic cane sugar or palm sugar
- Two lemons, zested and juiced
- One cup of basil leaves, packed
- Pinch salt

Directions:

1. In a small saucepan, bring the water and sugar to a boil. When the water is boiling, add the lemon zest, basil leaves, and salt. Remove from the heat and cover with a lid. For at least 20 minutes, steep the basil leaves in the simple syrup.
2. Meanwhile, fill a 4-cup measuring pitcher halfway with lemon juice. Juice the grapefruits into the pitcher until 3 glasses of combined juices are measured.
3. Remove the basil leaves and strain the simple syrup. Then combine the syrup and the juice. Refrigerate for at least 2-3 hours (or to speed up, put in the freezer for 1 hour.)
4. Fill an electric ice cream maker halfway with the sorbet mixture. Turn on and mix for at least 20 minutes, or until the mixture achieves a "soft-serve" consistency.

5.	Sorbet may be eaten right away or frozen in an airtight container. Allow the sorbet to soften for 10-15 minutes after it has been frozen before serving.

Note: to achieve the brightest, freshest flavor, use freshly squeezed grapefruits rather than pre-squeezed grapefruit juice.

Nutrition facts: calories: 272 | carbohydrates: 70 g | protein: 1 g | fat: 1 g | cholesterol: 38 mg

130. Bruleed grapefruit (pamplemousse brûlé)

Preparation Time: 5 minutes
Cooking Time: 8 minutes
Total time: 13 minutes
Servings: 8

Ingredients:
- 4 large ripe ruby red grapefruits
- 8 teaspoons granulated sugar
- Brulee torch

Directions:
1.	Place your index finger on the top of a grapefruit stem and cup your palm around it from top to bottom. Then, cut it in half in the middle. (if you don't notice a floral pattern, you've chopped the grapefruit the incorrect way.) Cut each grapefruit in this manner.
2.	I am using a tiny serrated knife cut along the inside rim of each grapefruit half to separate the fruit from the skin. Then, cut along the membrane between each small triangle section so that each mouthful comes out easily with a spoon. Keep everything intact.
3.	Sprinkle 1 teaspoon of granulated sugar over the top of each grapefruit half, one at a time. Then, hold the flame over the grapefruit and brulee the top until the sugar turns golden and has candied the top of each half. This should take 30-60 seconds per half. Serve immediately and repeat.

Nutrition facts: calories: 67 | carbohydrates: 12 g | protein: 2 g | fat: 2 g | cholesterol: 86 mg

131. Frozen beeritas recipe

Preparation Time: 5 minutes
Cooking Time: 5 minutes
Total time: 10 minutes

Servings: 2

Ingredients:
- 3 oz tequila blanco
- Oz triple sec (orange liqueur)
- 3 oz fresh lime juice
- 3 oz simple syrup
- 2 oz orange juice
- 14 oz mexican beer, such as two 7-ounce coronitas or one 12-ounce can any mexican beer
- 3-4 cups ice

Directions:
Self-serve method
1.	In a blender, combine tequila, triple sec, lime juice, simple syrup, and orange juice. Pour with 3 glasses of ice. Puree the mixture until it is smooth and foamy. Serve the margaritas in two big tumblers, with a coronita on the side. As they sip their margarita, each individual can add beer to it.
Mixed batch method
2.	In a blender, combine the tequila, triple sec, lime juice, simple syrup, orange juice, and a 12-ounce lager. Pour with 4 glasses of ice. Puree the mixture until it is smooth and foamy. Pour into serving glasses and serve.

Nutrition facts: calories: 386 | carbohydrates: 51 g | protein: 1 g | fat: 0 g | cholesterol: 55 mg

132. Spicy pineapple habanero margaritas

Preparation Time: 5 minutes
Cooking Time: 5 minutes
Total time: 10 minutes
Servings: 6

Ingredients:
- 1 cup tequila silver
- 1 cup triple sec
- 1 cup fresh-squeezed lime juice
- 2 1/2 cups pineapple juice
- 4 habanero chiles
- Optional garnishes: salt, limes, habaneros, pineapple slices

Directions:
1.	Melt the butter in a small pan over medium heat. Remove the from the habaneros by cutting them in half. Place the chiles in the skillet and cook

until they are blistered on both sides. Remove from the heat.

2.   In a pitcher, combine the tequila, triple sec, lime juice, and pineapple juice. Stir everything together thoroughly.

3.   Toss in the blistered habaneros. Allow them to soak in the margarita mix for 15 minutes to overnight. The longer they soak in the mixture, the hotter it will get. After 15 minutes, taste the mixture to see how long you want to soak them. When the heat level is to your taste, remove the habaneros.

4.   Pour the margaritas into glasses with ice when ready to serve. Garnish with lime wedges, pineapple slices, or more habaneros if desired.

Nutrition facts: calories: 287 | carbohydrates: 31 g | protein: 1 g | fat: 0 g | cholesterol: 65 mg

133. Cranberry pomegranate margarita with spiced rim

Preparation Time: 5 minutes
Cooking Time: 5 minutes
Total time: 10 minutes
Servings: 4

Ingredients:
- 2 cups cranberry pomegranate juice blend
- 2 cups tequila blanco
- 1 cup fresh squeezed lime juice
- 1/2 cup triple sec
- 2 tablespoons coarse sea salt
- 1 teaspoon old el paso taco seasoning
- 2 tablespoons agave syrup

Directions:
1.   1 tablespoon water and 1 tablespoon agave syrup on a dish to combine, gently mix everything together.
2.   On a separate dish, combine the salt and old el paso taco seasoning.
3.   Using the agave syrup, coat the rims of 4-6 glasses. Then, dip the rims in the seasoned salt. Fill the cups halfway with ice.
4.   In a large ice-filled shaker or pitcher, combine the cranberry pomegranate juice, tequila, lime juice, and triple sec. Shake or mix before pouring into glasses and serving!

Nutrition facts: calories: 483 | carbohydrates: 38 g | protein: 0 g | fat: 0 g | cholesterol: 346 mg

134. Peach milkshake (copycat chik-fil-a peach shake recipe!)

Preparation Time: 5 minutes
Cooking Time: 5 minutes
Total time: 10 minutes
Servings: 4

Ingredients:
- 6 ripe peaches pitted, skins on
- 7 scoops of vanilla ice cream
- 3 tablespoons granulated sugar
- ½ teaspoon vanilla extract
- 1 pinch salt
- Optional: whipped cream and maraschino cherries

Directions:
1.   Remove the pits from the peaches and cut them in half.
2.   Combine the peaches, ice cream, sugar, vanilla, and salt in a large blender.
3.   Puree till smooth, covered.

Nutrition facts: calories: 397 | carbohydrates: 62 g | protein: 7 g | fat: 9 g | cholesterol: 14 mg

135. Jugo verde (green juice)

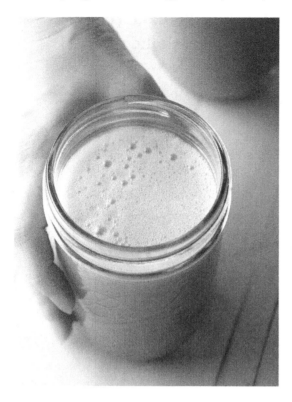

Preparation Time: 10 minutes
Cooking Time: 0 minutes
Total time: 10 minutes
Servings: 5

Ingredients:
- 2 cups orange juice
- 1 1/2 cups fresh pineapple chunks
- 1/2 nopal cactus paddle chopped (or substitute 1 celery stalk)
- 1 large cucumber with peel, cut into chunks
- 1/4 cup packed parsley or cilantro

Directions:
1. In a blender, combine all of the ingredients. Add a bit of salt, close the lid tightly, and puree until smooth.
2. When the mixture is green and frothy, serve immediately or strain over a screen to remove the pulp.

Nutrition facts: calories: 67 | carbohydrates: 12 g | protein: 2 g | fat: 2 g | cholesterol: 86 mg

136. Perfect manhattan recipe

Preparation Time: 2 minutes
Cooking Time: 5 minutes
Total time: 7 minutes
Servings: 1

Ingredients:
- 2 oz bourbon or rye whiskey
- 1-ounce sweet vermouth like antica
- 2 dashes of angostura bitters
- Garnishes: twist of lemon rind, orange rind, or a maraschino cherry

Directions:
1. Fill a cocktail shaker halfway with ice for each manhattan cocktail. Combine the bourbon, sweet vermouth, and bitters in a mixing glass.
2. Using a bar spoon, stir everything together. Don't jiggle. Then strain into a coupe cocktail glass or a low ball glass filled with ice.
3. Serve with a maraschino cherry, lemon peel twist, or orange rind twist as a garnish.

Nutrition facts: calories: 190 | carbohydrates: 2 g | protein: 1 g | fat: 16 g | cholesterol: 293 mg

137. Frozen coconut mojito

Preparation Time: 5 minutes
Cooking Time: 5 minutes
Total time: 10 minutes
Servings: 2

Ingredients:
- 4 oz cream of coconut
- 4 oz coconut rum
- 2 oz fresh lime juice
- 8 fresh mint leaves
- 4 cups ice

Directions:
1. In a high-powered blender, combine all of the ingredients with 4 cups of ice. Pour into glasses after blending until totally smooth.
2. If desired, garnish with mint and lime slices.

Nutrition facts: calories: 386 | carbohydrates: 43 g | protein: 1 g | fat: 9 g | cholesterol: 182 mg

138. Mulled lemonade recipe

Preparation Time: 20 minutes
Cooking Time: 5 minutes
Total time: 25 minutes
Servings: 8

Ingredients:

- 5 cups water divided
- 1 cup granulated sugar
- 1 cup fresh lemon juice
- 3 cinnamon sticks
- 6 whole star anise
- 4 slices fresh ginger
- 4 pieces orange peel large
- 20 whole cloves
- 6 cracked green cardamom pods
- 1/2 teaspoon pink peppercorns

Directions:

1.   2 cups of water, brought to a boil mix in the sugar and all of the pieces. Allow the simple syrup to steep for at least 20 minutes, covered. (the more time you have, the better.)

2.   Fill a big pitcher halfway with syrup. Then add the remaining three cups of water and lemon juice. Fill the pitcher halfway with ice and swirl well.
Notes: if you don't want "floaties" in your drinks, drain the spices out of the simple syrup.

Nutrition facts: calories: 117 | carbohydrates: 30 g | protein: 1 g | fat: 1 g | cholesterol: 70 mg

139. Cucumber rose aperol spritz
Preparation Time: 5 minutes
Cooking Time: 5 minutes
Total time: 10 minutes
Servings: 1

Ingredients:

- Oz rose-infused aperol*
- 2 oz sparkling wine such as prosecco
- 2 slices cucumber about an inch thick
- Splash club soda

Directions:

1.   To make rose-infused aperol, mix one 750ml bottle aperol with one ounce dried rose petals (these can be found in the bulk section of most specialty food stores). Shake everything together and set it aside for a few hours or overnight. After straining off the rose petals, the aperol is ready to use.

2.   In a cocktail shaker, combine the rose aperol and cucumber with ice. Fill a tall collins glass halfway with ice and strain it into it. Pour in the sparkling wine and ice. Garnish with fresh cucumber and a dash of club soda.

Nutrition facts: calories: 143 | carbohydrates: 12 g | protein: 1 g | fat: 1 g | cholesterol: 50 mg

140. Pink grapefruit margarita
Preparation Time: 5 minutes
Cooking Time: 0 minutes
Total time: 5 minutes
Servings: 2

Ingredients:

- Five oz of freshly squeezed ruby red grapefruit juice
- Four oz of white tequila
- 1 1/2 oz of triple sec orange liquor
- 1/2 ounce of agave syrup + extra for glass rims
- Fresh grapefruit slices for garnish
- Salt for rim

Directions:

1.   Put a little quantity of agave syrup on one plate and salt on another. Dip the rims of the glasses first in the syrup, then in the salt. Fill the cups halfway with ice and set them aside.

2.   Fill an ice-filled cocktail shaker halfway with ice. Fill the shaker halfway with fresh grapefruit juice, tequila, triple sec, and agave.

3.   Cover and vigorously shake for 30 seconds. After that, pour into the glasses. Enjoy with fresh grapefruit slices as a garnish!

Nutrition facts: calories: 251 | carbohydrates: 20 g | protein: 1 g | fat: 1 g | cholesterol: 192 mg

141. Strawberry margarita recipe
Preparation Time: 10 minutes
Cooking Time: 0 minutes
Total time: 10 minutes
Servings: 2

Ingredients:

- 1 pound fresh strawberries, trimmed
- 1 cup tequila
- 3/4 cup fresh lime juice
- 2/3 cup strawberry jam
- 1/4 cup triple sec
- 10 mint leaves

- 3-4 cups ice
- Optional garnish: margarita salt, lime slices, extra strawberries

Directions:
1. Prepare a big blender. Add the fresh-cut strawberries, tequila, lime juice, strawberry jam, triple sec, mint leaves, and ice to the container.
2. Blend until smooth.
3. Toppings: paint additional strawberry jam around the rims of four glasses using a pastry brush. Dip the rims of the glasses in margarita salt.
4. Fill the glass halfway with cold margaritas. Serve with a fresh lime slice and a strawberry on top.

Nutrition facts: calories: 391 | carbohydrates: 57 g | protein: 1 g | fat: 1 g | cholesterol: 142 mg

142. Large-batch goombay smash caribbean cocktails

Preparation Time: 5 minutes
Cooking Time: 3 minutes
Total time: 8 minutes
Servings: 40

Ingredients:
- 14 cups 100% pineapple juice
- 2 bottles of dark caribbean rum (750 ml each - i used pusser's)
- 1 bottle coconut rum (750 ml - cruzan)
- 2 cups fresh-squeezed lime juice
- 1 1/2 cups simple syrup
- 1 cup orange liqueur (cointreau)
- 1/2 teaspoon bitters, optional
- Fresh pineapple slices for garnish

Directions:
1. If you're creating your own simple syrup, mix 1 cup granulated sugar and 1 cup water. Cook until the sugar melts on the burner. Allow cooling fully.
2. Fill a big beverage dispenser halfway with all of the ingredients. Stir everything together thoroughly. Chill until ready to serve, then top with cut pineapples.
3. Serve with ice.

Nutrition facts: calories: 222 | carbohydrates: 22 g | protein: 0 g | fat: 0 g | cholesterol: 11 mg

143. Healthy vegan brownies

Preparation Time: 15 minutes
Cooking Time: 30 minutes
Total time: 45 minutes
Servings: 9

Ingredients:
- 4 tablespoon ground flax
- ⅔ cup warm water
- 1 cup date sugar or coconut sugar
- 1 cup cacao powder
- ½ cup white whole wheat flour
- ½ tablespoon salt
- 1 tablespoon baking powder
- ½ cup unsweetened applesauce or pumpkin puree
- 1 tablespoon vanilla extract
- ¼ cup unsweetened almond milk optional

Directions:
6. Preheat the oven to 325 degrees fahrenheit. In a small dish, combine ground flax and warm water. Allow for a 15-minute resting period.
7. In a medium mixing bowl, combine the dry ingredients (date sugar, cacao powder, white whole wheat flour, baking powder, and salt) while the flax egg is setting.
8. In the middle of the dry ingredients, make a well. Combine the wet and dry components (flax egg, applesauce/or pumpkin puree, and vanilla extract). Stir until well mixed. If the batter appears to be too dry, add 14 cups of unsweetened almond milk.
9. Pour the batter into an 8-inch square baking dish lined with parchment paper. Distribute evenly.
10. 30–35 minutes in the oven, or until a toothpick inserted in the middle comes out clean. Allow cooling fully in the pan before removing and cutting into squares.

Nutrition facts: calories: 126 | carbohydrates: 28 g | protein: 3 g | fat: 1 g | cholesterol: 172 mg

144. Green chicken soup

Preparation Time: 15 minutes
Cooking Time: 25 minutes
Total time: 40 minutes
Servings: 12

Ingredients:
- Two quarts of chicken broth or stock
- 1 ½ pound boneless, skinless chicken breast

- Two celery stalks, chopped
- Two cups of green beans, cut into 1-inch pieces
- One and a half cups peas, fresh or frozen
- Two cups asparagus, cut into 1-inch pieces, tops and middles (avoid tough ends)
- One cup of diced green onions
- 4-6 cloves garlic, minced
- Two cups of fresh spinach leaves, chopped and packed
- One bunch watercress, chopped with large stems removed
- 1/2 cup of fresh parsley leaves, chopped
- 1/3 cup of fresh basil leaves, chopped
- One teaspoon salt

Directions:

1. In a large saucepan, boil the chicken broth over medium-high heat. Bring the chicken breasts to a simmer in the sauce. The cooking time is 15 minutes.
2. Combine the celery, green beans, peas, asparagus, onions, garlic, salt in a mixing bowl. Simmer for 5-10 minutes, or until the vegetables are soft, then remove from the heat.
3. Remove the chicken breasts and shred or cut them into bite-sized pieces with two forks. Back to the pot.
4. Combine the spinach, watercress, parsley, and basil in a mixing bowl. Season with salt to taste.

Nutrition facts: calories: 105 | carbohydrates: 7 g | protein: 15 g | fat: 2 g | cholesterol: 134 mg

145. Green risotto recipe

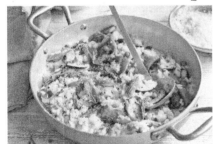

Preparation Time: 10 minutes
Cooking Time: 40 minutes
Total time: 50 minutes
Servings: 8

Ingredients:
- Two cups arborio rice
- Three tablespoons butter
- Three tablespoons olive oil
- Six scallions, greens and whites chopped
- Two and a half cups fresh packed spinach leaves
- One cup packed fresh parsley
- 12 fresh basil leaves
- Three garlic cloves
- Six cups chicken broth, room temperature (vegetable broth for vegetarians)
- One cup of white wine
- One cup of shredded parmesan cheese
- Salt

Directions:

1. In a blender, combine spinach, parsley, basil, and garlic. Add 4 cups broth and purée until completely smooth.
2. In a large sauté pan, combine the butter and oil. In a medium saucepan over medium heat, melt the butter. Add the scallions once the butter has melted and cooked for 2 minutes. After adding the rice, cook for another 2 minutes. Then stir in the wine, 1 1/2 teaspoons of salt, and 1/2 teaspoon ground.
3. Simmer, occasionally stirring, until the wine has been absorbed. Start with the 2 cups of liquid that was not put into the blender and add one cup of broth at a time to the rice. Stir the rice after each addition of liquid and let it boil until the broth is absorbed before adding more. Ensure that all of the green herb broth is included in the blender. This procedure will take approximately 25 minutes.
4. Stir in the grated parmesan cheese after you've poured the rest of the green liquid and the rice is cooked but still firm. Turn off the heat before the last round of stock has been completely absorbed, leaving the risotto a bit soupy. As it cools, it will stiffen up. Season to taste with salt and serve warm.

Nutrition facts: calories: 283 | carbohydrates: 36 g | protein: 1 g | fat: 1 g | cholesterol: 53 mg

Chapter 11. Lunch low fiber

146. Barbecue Beef Stir-Fry

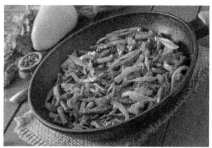

Preparation time: 5 minutes
Cooking time: 25 minutes
Servings: 4
Ingredients:

- Barbecue Sauce – ¼ cup
- Beef broth – three tbsp, low-sodium
- Beef sirloin steak – one lb, boneless, cut into strips
- Onion – one, sliced
- Carrot – one, thinly sliced
- Oil – one tablespoon
- Hot cooked long-grain white rice – two cups

Directions:

1. Combine the broth and BBQ sauce into the bowl.
2. Rub one tbsp of meat and let stand for five minutes.
3. Add vegetable, meat, and oil into the skillet and cook over medium-high flame for four minutes.
4. Add remaining BBQ sauce mixture and combine well. Let simmer over medium-low flame for two minutes.

Serve and enjoy!
Nutrition:
Calories;   310kcal,   carbohydrates; 34g, protein; 23g, fat; 9g

147. Chicken Saffron Rice Pilaf

Preparation time: 15 minutes
Cooking time: 30 minutes
Serving: 6
Ingredients:

- Saffron – one pinch
- Ghee or olive oil – one tbsp
- Carrot – one, peeled, chopped
- Celery – one stalk, outside parts peeled, chopped
- Basmati rice or jasmine rice – 1 ½ cups
- Chicken broth – three cups, low-sodium
- Chicken breast – 1 ¼ cups, roasted, shredded
- Lemon – one
- Fresh parsley – chopped, to garnish

Directions:

1. Add saffron and water into the bowl and soak it.
2. Add ghee into the skillet and heat it. Then, add celery and carrots and sauté for three to four minutes until softened. Add rice and sauté until toasted.
3. Add saffron and chicken broth to the skillet, bring to a boil, lower the heat, and cook for twenty-five to thirty minutes.
4. Add shredded chicken to the rice and toss to combine.
5. Let sit for five minutes.
6. When ready to serve, add lemon juice over the rice.
7. Garnish with chopped parsley leaves.

Nutrition:
Calories; 269kcal, Carbohydrates; 41g, Fats; 5g Proteins; 13g

148. Stir-Fry Ground Chicken and Green Beans

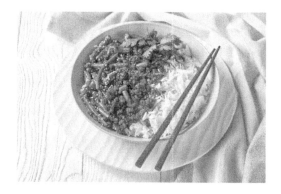

Preparation time: 5 minutes
Cooking time: 5-10 minutes
Serving: 2
Ingredients:

- Green bean – 2 cups
- Oil – one tbsp
- Ginger – one slice
- Ground chicken – ½ lb

- Soy sauce – 1 tbsp
- Rice wine – 1 tsp
- Sesame oil – 1 tsp
- Sugar – 1 tsp

Directions:
1. Add green beans into the boiled water and cook until tender.
2. Drain it and put it into the bowl of ice water.
3. Add oil into the skillet and heat it. Then, add a ginger slice and fry for one to two minutes.
4. Add ground chicken and cook until no longer pink.
5. Add sugar, sesame oil, rice wine, and soy sauce and toss to combine.
6. Add drained green beans and cook them.
7. Serve and enjoy!

Nutrition:
Calories; 162kcal, Carbohydrates; 10g, Fats; 18g Proteins; 22g, fiber; 2g

149. Stewed Lamb

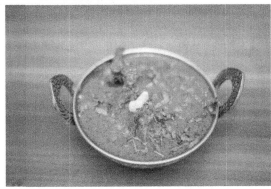

Preparation time: 5 minutes
Cooking time: 8 hours
Serving: 6
Ingredients:
- Lamb leg – 1 1/2kg, boneless
- Extra-virgin olive oil – 2 tbsp
- Beef or vegetable broth – 400ml
- Red wine – 300ml
- Wholemeal flour – 80g
- Button mushrooms – 400g, sliced in half
- Fresh rosemary leaves – 1 tsp
- Potatoes – 1kg, cut into quarters, red-skinned
- Celery sticks – two chopped
- Carrots – two, cut into large chunks

Parsley – 1 cup, chopped

Directions:
1. Add olive oil into the saucepan and place it over medium flame.
2. Cook until browned. Add stock to the slow cooker, place the lamb with all ingredients into the slow cooker, and cook on low flame for eight hours.
3. After eight hours, turn off the slow cooker and add cooled stock to the bowl to make a paste with wholemeal flour. Stir well.
4. Add flour paste and sprinkle with pepper and salt.
5. Sprinkle with fresh parsley leaves.

Nutrition:
Calories; 481kcal, Carbohydrates; 22g, Fats; 27g Proteins; 28g, fiber; 4g

150. Pulled Chicken Salad

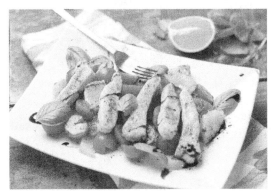

Preparation time: 5 minutes
Cooking time: 5 minutes
Serving: 4
Ingredients:
Pulled BBQ chicken – 200g, cooked
- Apricots – 1/3 cup, drained, thinly sliced
- Orzo pasta – 100g
- Spinach – 150g, stalks removed
- Cheddar cheese, 70g, cut into small cubes
- Parmesan cheese – 30g
- Parsley – ¼ cup, chopped
- Noodles – 1/3 cup
- Olive oil – five tbsp
- Red wine vinegar – three tbsp
- Salt and pepper, to taste

Directions:
1. Shred cooked and cooled chicken with a fork.

2. Add cooked and cooled orzo pasta into the microwave dish. Top with parmesan cheese and microwave for one to two minutes.
3. Add apricots, chicken, parsley, and spinach into the bowl and mix it well. Then, add red wine vinegar and olive oil, sprinkle with pepper and salt, and pour over the salad. Combine it well.
4. Add crispy noodles before serving.

Nutrition:
Calories; 352kcal, Carbohydrates; 14g, Fats; 19g Proteins; 29g, fiber; 3g

151. Lemongrass Beef

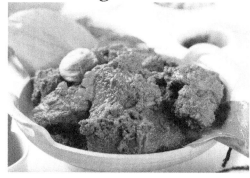

Preparation time: 5 minutes
Cooking time: 5-10 minutes
Serving: 4
Ingredients:

- Sesame oil – 2 tbsp
- Fish sauce – 1 tbsp
- Sweet chili sauce – 2 tbsp
- Basmati rice – 2 packets, microwave
- Coconut – 2 tsp, shredded
- Lemongrass paste – 1 tbsp
- Beef – 500g, minced, grass-fed
- Thai seasoning – 1 tbsp
- Cucumber – 100g, peeled and cut into chunks
- Carrots – two, peeled and julienned
- Basil – ¼ cup, chopped
- Lime – one, cut into four wedges

Directions:
1. Add sesame oil, lemongrass paste, fish sauce, and Thai seasoning into the wok and heat it. Add the minced beef and stir well and cook for three to four minutes until browned.
2. Cook the rice according to the instructions.
3. Add one tsp shredded coconut and stir well.

4. Add carrots, cucumber, rice, and minced beef into the bowl.
5. Sprinkle with Thai basil.
6. Pour sweet chili sauce and lime wedges over it.

Nutrition:
Calories; 450kcal, Carbohydrates; 50g, Fats; 19g Proteins; 21g, fiber; 3g

152. Beetroot Carrot Salad

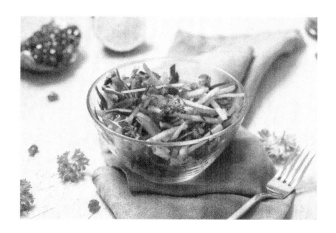

Preparation time: 5 minutes
Cooking time: 40 minutes
Serving: 6
Ingredients:

- Beetroot – three, peeled
- Carrots – three, peeled
- Halloumi, 500g, thickly sliced
- Fresh oregano leaves – one tsp
- Maple syrup – 100ml
- Fresh lemon juice – 50ml
- Spinach leaves – 50g
- Tahini – 200g, hulled
- Noodles – 100g
- Extra virgin olive oil – 2 tbsp

Directions:
1. Preheat the oven to 180 degrees C.
2. Wrap the beetroot and carrots into the foil and put it into the oven for forty minutes.
3. Let cool it and then cut into the wedges.
4. Add olive oil into the saucepan and place it over medium flame.
5. Turn off the flame and add oregano, lemon juice, and maple syrup and stir well.
6. Add one tbsp of hulled tahini onto the plate.
7. Top with beetroot and carrot wedges, halloumi and spinach leaves.

8. Sprinkle with crispy noodles.

Nutrition:
Calories; 206kcal, Carbohydrates; 34.9g, Fats; 6.6g Proteins; 4.5g, fiber; 4g

153. Crunchy Maple Sweet Potatoes

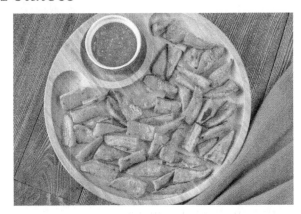

Preparation time: 5 minutes
Cooking time: 30 minutes
Serving: 4
Ingredients:

- Allspice – one pinch
- Pure maple syrup – 2 tbsp
- Cashew nuts – ¼ cup, crushed
- **Potatoes:**
- Extra-virgin olive oil spray
- White potatoes – 500g, peeled
- Sweet potato – one, peeled
- Plain white flour – ¼ cup
- Apple juice – ½ cup
- Butter – one tbsp
- Sweet soy sauce – 1 tsp
- Maple syrup – one tbsp
- Cinnamon – one pinch
- Salt and pepper – to taste

Directions:

1. Preheat the oven to 180 degrees C.
2. Mix all ingredients into the dish, place it into the oven, and bake for ten to fifteen minutes until golden and crunchy.
3. Keep it aside.
4. **Potatoes:**
5. Let boil the potatoes for fifteen to twenty minutes.
6. Spray the baking dish with extra virgin olive oil.

7. Slice potatoes into chunks and place them onto the dish.
8. Add all other ingredients into the bowl and combine them well.
9. Pour mixture over the potatoes and cover with a lid and bake for ten minutes.
10. Sprinkle with nuts.

Nutrition:
Calories; 92kcal, Carbohydrates; 18g, Fats; 2g Proteins; 1.2g, fiber; 1g

154. Veggie Bowl

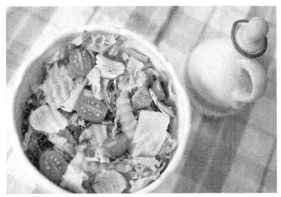

Preparation time: 10 minutes
Serving: 2
Ingredients:

- White basmati rice – 100g
- Green beans – six
- Red pepper, peeled, diced, and roasted
- Ripe avocado – ¼, sliced lengthways
- Cucumber – half cup, sliced
- Asparagus – six stems
- Tuna – one slice
- Pumpkin chunks – ½ cup, peeled and roasted
- Lemon – half, cut into quarters
- Ginger – 2 tsp, pickled
- **Dressing:**
- Orange juice – ½ cup, freshly squeezed
- Sesame oil – four tbsp
- Salt and pepper, one pinch

Directions:

1. Cook the rice and drain it well.
2. Blanche green beans.
3. Grill red pepper and remove skin and then dice it.
4. Thinly slice the avocado lengthways.
5. Cut the cucumber thinly.

6. Drain six stems of asparagus.
7. Drain tuna slices of oil.
8. Boil the pumpkin chunks.
9. Place the red pepper in a mound in the middle of the plates.
10. Arrange all ingredients on the plates.
11. Pour sesame oil over it. Sprinkle with pepper and salt.
12. Pour dressing over the bowl.

Nutrition:
Calories; 519kcal, Carbohydrates; 59.2g, Fats; 28.4g Proteins; 13.2g, fiber; 5g

155. Pomegranate Salad

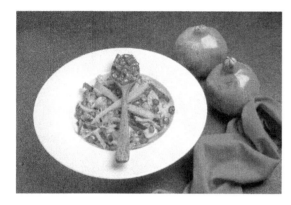

Preparation time: 5 minutes
Cooking time: 10 minutes
Serving: 4
Ingredients:

- Chives – one tsp, chopped
- Zucchini – 300g
- Baby spinach – 100g
- Red pepper – one, skinned
- Extra-virgin olive oil spray
- **Dressing:**
- Walnut oil – three tbsp
- Pomegranate juice – ¼ cup
- Dijon mustard – 2 tsp
- Salt – to taste

Directions:
1. Add all ingredients into the bowl and beat until combined for dressing.
2. Slice zucchini into chunks. Let chop the chives.
3. Spray the zucchini and chives with olive oil.
4. Place a frypan over medium flame.
5. Add chives and zucchini and fry until golden brown.
6. Then, add baby spinach leaves and stir well.

7. Turn off the flame. Pour dressing over the salad.

Nutrition:
Calories; 273kcal, Carbohydrates; 14.9g, Fats; 21.4g Proteins; 9.5g, fiber; 2g

156. Dijon Orange Summer Salad

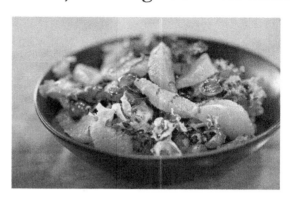

Preparation time: 10 minutes
Serving: 2
Ingredients:

- Baby spinach leaves – 150g
- Oranges – two, peeled, deseeded and sliced thinly
- Crushed macadamia nuts – 60g
- Feta cheese – 100g
- **Dressing:**
- Thyme leaves – 1 tbsp
- Extra-virgin olive oil – 4 tbsp
- Dijon mustard – 1 tbsp
- Lemon juice – 4 tbsp
- Sourdough white bread rolls – 2 crusty

Directions:
1. Add salad ingredients into the bowl.
2. Add dressing ingredients into the jar and shake it well.
3. Pour dressing over the salad. Combine it well.
4. Serve with a sourdough white bread roll.

Nutrition:
Calories; 27kcal, Carbohydrates; 6.7g, Proteins; 0.2g, fiber; 3g

157. Pulao Rice Prawns

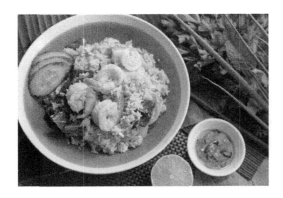

Preparation time: 5 minutes
Cooking time: 10 minutes
Serving: 4
Ingredients:
Prawns – 20, deveined, shelled

- Extra virgin olive oil – three tbsp
- Water – 500ml
- Coconut milk – 200ml
- Cardamoms – three
- Bay leaves – two
- Red chili powder – one pinch
- Turmeric powder – ½ tsp
- Fresh coriander – ¼ cup, chopped
- Black pepper and pepper – to taste
- Garam masala powder – one pinch
- Asafoetida powder – one pinch

Directions:
1. Add olive oil into the pan. Heat it. Then, add black pepper, cardamoms, bay leaves, and spices clove and cook for one to two minutes until fragrant, about one to two minutes.
2. Add cardamom, bay leaves, and cloves into the tea leaf ball.
3. Add asafoetida powder, turmeric, garam masala, chili powder, salt, and prawns and combine well. Drain and add rice to the pan and cover with 500ml water and 200ml coconut milk.
4. Lower the heat and simmer until cooked thoroughly.
5. Garnish with fresh coriander leaves.

Nutrition:
Calories; 424kcal, Carbohydrates; 62g, Fats; 11g Proteins; 19g, fiber; 2g

158. White Radish Crunch Salad

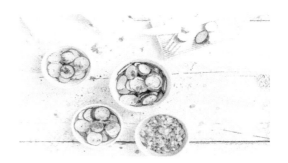

Preparation time: 5 minutes
Serving: 2
Ingredients:
Radish – 200g, julienned

- Cucumber – 200g, shredded
- Noodles – 50g
- Ginger – 1 tsp, grated, steamed
- Nori – ¼ sheet, thinly sliced
- **Dressing:**
- Soy sauce – 1 tsp
- Rice vinegar – 1 tsp
- Maple syrup – 1 tsp
- Orange juice – 1 tbsp
- Sesame oil – 1 tbsp

Directions:
1. Combine cucumber, ginger, and radish into the bowl. Pour dressing ingredients over it. Top with nori and noodles. Stir well.
2. Serve!

Nutrition:
Calories; 82kcal, Carbohydrates; 5g, Fats; 7g Proteins; 1g, fiber; 2g

159. Apple and mushroom Soup

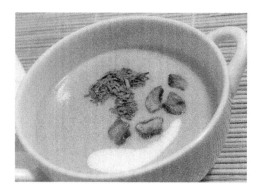

Preparation time: 5 minutes
Cooking time: 5 minutes
Serving: 2
Ingredients:

- Water – 400ml
- Green apple – half, peeled, cored and grated
- Precooked rice noodles – 100g
- Green chives – ¼ cup, chopped
- Mushrooms – 2, sliced
- Silken tofu – 100g, crumbed
- Roasted seaweed – 1 slice

Directions:

1. Rinse the rice noodles in hot water and then strain them.
2. Add all ingredients and stir for one to two minutes.
3. Then, add crushed seaweed flakes.
4. Serve!

Nutrition:
Calories; 366kcal, Carbohydrates; 41.1g, Fats; 19g Proteins; 11g, Fibers; 3g

160. Spring Watercress Soup

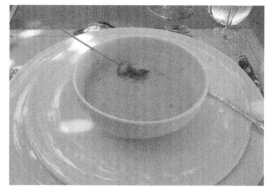

Preparation time: 5 minutes

Cooking time: 20-25 minutes
Serving: 4
Ingredients:

- Watercress – one bunch, rinsed
- Olive oil – 1 tbsp
- Green onion – 1, diced, green part only
- Chicken stock – four cups
- Baby arugula – four cups
- Sea salt – to taste
- Chives – 1 tbsp, snipped
- Greek yogurt – 2 tbsp

Directions:

1. Separate the thick and tough stems from the watercress leaves.
2. Dice the stems. Reserve the leaves.
3. Add oil to the pot or Dutch oven and place it over medium-high flame.
4. Then, add the green onion (green part only) and diced watercress stems into the pot, lower the heat to medium, and sprinkle with salt.
5. Cook for five minutes.
6. Add stock and bring to a boil over medium-high flame.
7. When boiled, lower the heat to medium-low and simmer for fifteen minutes.
8. Add reserved watercress leaves and arugula and cook until wilted.
9. Turn off the flame.
10. Add soup into the immersion blender and blend until smooth.
11. Place soup back in the pan/pot and warm through.
12. Garnish with chopped chives.

Nutrition:
Calories; 174kcal, Carbohydrates; 19g, Fats; 7g Proteins; 10g

161. Oyster Sauce Tofu

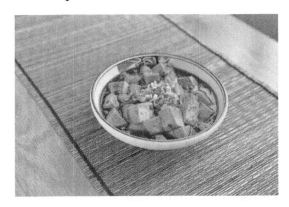

Preparation time: 10 minutes
Cooking time: 15 minutes
Serving: 4
Ingredients:
- Tofu – 700g
- Oil – 2 tsp
- Ginger – one slice, peeled, minced
- Scallion – one, trimmed, chopped
- Chicken broth or vegetable broth – 1 ½ cups, low sodium
- Oyster sauce – three tbsp
- Rice wine – 2 tsp
- Cornstarch – 2 tsp
- Water – 1 tsp
- Sesame oil – 1 tsp

Directions:
1. Slice tofu into bite-sized squares and keep it aside.
2. Add oil into the skillet and heat it.
3. Then, add ginger and green part of chopped scallions and cook for one to two minutes.
4. Add tofu, rice wine, broth, and oyster sauce and bring to a boil.
5. Lower the heat and to medium-low and simmer for five minutes.
6. Add water and cornstarch into the bowl and stir to make a slurry.
7. Add tofu into the gravy and drizzle with sesame oil, and sprinkle with green parts of scallions.

Nutrition:
Calories; 58kcal, Carbohydrates; 4g, Fats; 3g Proteins; 2g

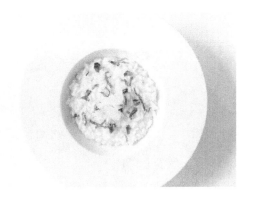

Preparation time: 10 minutes
Cooking time: 30 minutes
Serving: 3
Ingredients:
- Olive oil – 2 tbsp
- Rosemary – 1 sprig, chopped
- Green onion – 1, diced, green part only
- Arborio rice – 2/3 cup
- Yukon gold potato – 1, rinsed, peeled scrubbed, diced
- Chicken stock – 3 ½ cups, low-sodium
- Parmesan cheese – 1 tbsp, grated
- Butter – 1 tsp
- Salt and pepper, to taste

Directions:
1. Add olive oil into the Dutch oven and heat it over medium-high flame.
2. Add rosemary and cook for one minute. Then, add green onion and cook for two minutes until translucent.
3. Turn the heat down to medium and sprinkle with salt. Let sweat for eight minutes.
4. Remove the lid and elevate the heat to medium-high and then add rice to it. Combine it well.
5. Add potato and cook for one minute more.
6. Add chicken stock and bring to a boil.
7. Lower the heat to low and simmer for twenty minutes until al dente.
8. Add butter and parmesan cheese and turn off the flame.
9. Let sit for five minutes.
10. Add more stock if needed.
11. Sprinkle with black pepper.

Nutrition:
Calories; 377kcal, Carbohydrates; 55g, Fats; 13g Proteins; 12g

162. Potato and Rosemary Risotto

163. Cheesy Baked Tortillas

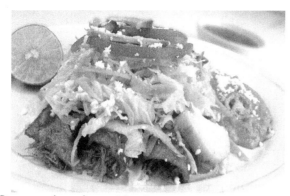

Preparation time: 10 minutes
Cooking time: 40 minutes
Serving: 4
Ingredients:

- Pizza sauce – 255g
- Extra-virgin olive oil – 20ml
- Extra-virgin olive oil spray
- Plain Greek yoghurt – as needed
- Juice of whole lime – one
- Onion powder – 1 tsp
- Sweet paprika – ½ tsp
- Cheddar cheese – 250g, low-fat
- Chicken – 250g, cooked, shredded
- White potato – 400g, peeled
- Basmati rice – 400g, cooked and drained
- Salt and pepper – to taste
- Flour tortillas – six

Directions:

1. Preheat the oven to 210 degrees C.
2. Spray the potatoes with olive oil spray.
3. Sprinkle with paprika powder and place it into the oven and bake for 20 minutes.
4. Add onion powder and olive oil into the pan and heat it for one minute.
5. Add tofu or chicken, 180g of pizza sauce, pepper, salt, and lemon juice, and combine well.
6. Layout tortillas onto the clean surface and top with chicken or tofu mixture, rice, and baked potatoes and top with cheese.
7. Roll the burritos and place them onto the dish.
8. Top with remaining cheese and bake for 15 to 20 minutes.

Nutrition:
Calories; 389kcal, Carbohydrates; 31g, Fats; 20g Proteins; 22g, fiber; 4g

164. Smoky Rice

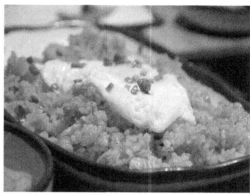

Preparation time: 10 minutes
Cooking time: 20 minutes
Serving: 4
Ingredients:

- White basmati rice – 400g
- Pasta – 200ml
- Green onion – half, peeled and chopped, green part only
- Red capsicum – ¼, chopped
- Extra-virgin olive oil – 4 tbsp
- Tomato puree – 70g
- Bay leaves – three
- Paprika – one tsp
- Cumin – one tsp
- Black pepper – one pinch
- Chili – one pinch
- Coconut oil – four tbsp
- Banana – peeled and chopped
- Salt – to taste

Directions:
Rice:

1. Rinse rice and soak for twenty minutes.
2. Let boil it for five minutes. Then, drain it.
3. Add black pepper, paprika, cumin, chili, half green onion (green part only), pasta, and red capsicum into the blender and blend until smooth.
4. Add oil into the saucepan and place it over medium flame.
5. Add capsicum mixture to the pan and sprinkle with salt and cook for few minutes until fragrant. Then, add tomato puree and bay leaves and cook for five minutes.
6. Add drained rice and one cup of water and simmer for eight minutes until the rice is soft. Discard bay leaves. Keep it aside.

Banana:
1. Add coconut oil and banana into the pan and cook until golden.
2. Add banana over the rice.
3. Serve!
4. **Nutrition:**

Calories; 447kcal, Carbohydrates; 69g, Fats; 11g Proteins; 11g, fiber; 3g

165. Zucchini Lasagna

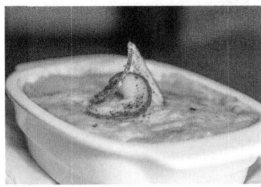

Preparation time: 10 minutes
Cooking time: 40 minutes
Serving: 4
Ingredients:

- Zucchini – 800g, grated
- Green onion – 1 tsp, green part only
- Chives – 1 tbsp, chopped
- Dried oregano – 1 tbsp
- Ricotta – 250g, low-fat
- Cheddar cheese – 50g, low-fat, shredded
- Passata – 350ml
- Dried lasagna sheets – nine, gluten-free
- Extra virgin oil – as needed
- Salt and pepper – to taste

Instruction:
Preheat the oven to 210 degrees C.
Add olive oil into the frying pan and heat it.
Add green onion and zucchini and cook for three minutes.
Lower the heat, add 25g of low-fat cheddar cheese and ricotta, and sprinkle with pepper and salt. Keep it aside.
Let boil the lasagna sheet in the salted water for five to six minutes.
Then, drain it. Add some olive oil to the pasta.
Place lasagna sheet onto the baking dish, add ricotta and zucchini mixture, and sprinkle with fresh chives and oregano. Then, add tomato pasata.

Lower the heat of the oven to 180 degrees C.
Bake the lasagna for thirty minutes.
Serve with salad.
Nutrition:
Calories; 362kcal, Carbohydrates; 7g, Fats; 26g Proteins; 25g, fiber; 3g

166. Greek Chicken Skewers

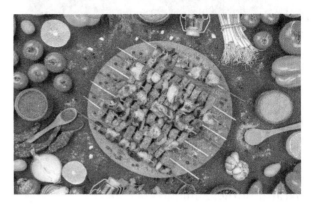

Preparation time: 20 minutes
Cooking time 20 minutes
Additional time: 2 hours
Servings: 4
Ingredients:

- Lemon juice – ¼ cup
- Wok oil – ¼ cup
- Red wine vinegar – 1/8 cup
- Onion flakes – one tbsp
- Garlic – one tbsp, minced
- Lemon – one, zested
- Greek seasoning – one tsp
- Poultry seasoning – one tsp
- Dried oregano – one tsp
- Ground black pepper – one tsp
- Dried thyme – half tsp
- Chicken breasts – three, cut into 1-inch pieces, skinless and boneless

Directions:
Whisk the thyme, pepper, oregano, poultry seasoning, Greek seasoning, lemon zest, garlic, onion flakes, vinegar, oil, and lemon juice into the bowl. Place it into the re-sealable plastic bag.
Add chicken and coat with marinade and seal the bag. Place it into the refrigerator for two hours.
Preheat the oven to 350 degrees Fahrenheit.
Discard marinade and thread chicken onto the skewers.
Place skewers onto the baking sheet.
Cook for twenty minutes until golden brown.

Nutrition:
Calories; 248kcal, carbohydrates; 4.1g, protein; 18.1g, fat; 17g

167. Roast Beef

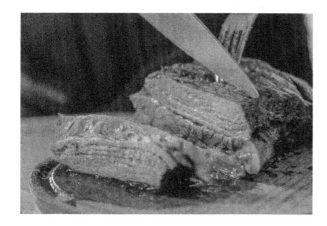

Preparation time: 5 minutes
Cooking time: 1 hour
Servings: 6
Ingredients:

- Beef eye of round roast – three pounds
- Kosher salt – half tsp
- Garlic powder – half tsp
- Freshly ground black pepper – ¼ tsp

Directions:

1. Preheat the oven to 375 degrees Fahrenheit.
2. Place roast into the pan and sprinkle with pepper, garlic powder, and salt. Cook it into the oven for one hour.
3. Let cool it for fifteen to twenty minutes.
4. Serve and enjoy!

Nutrition:
Calories; 48kcal, carbohydrates; 0.2g, protein; 44.8g, fat; 32.4g

168. Banana Cake

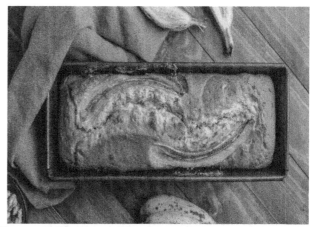

Preparation time: 20 minutes
Cooking time: 1 hour 15 minutes
Servings: 15
Ingredients:

- Bananas – 1 1/3 cup, mashed
- Lemon juice – 2 ½ tbsp
- Milk – 1 ½ cups
- Flour – three cups
- Baking soda – 1 ½ tsp
- Salt – ¼ tsp
- Butter – 2/3 cup, softened
- White sugar – one cup
- Brown sugar – half cup
- Eggs – three
- Vanilla – one tsp

Frosting:

- Cream cheese – eight ounces
- Butter – 1/3 cup, softened
- Powdered sugar – 3 ½ cups
- Lemon juice – one tsp
- 1 ½ tsp lemon zest from one lemon

Directions:

1. Preheat the oven to 350 degrees Fahrenheit. Grease and flour the pan.
2. Add 1 ½ tbsp lemon juice into the cup. Then, add one and a half cups milk and keep it aside.
3. Combine one tbsp lemon juice and mashed banana and keep it aside.
4. Add white sugar, brown sugar, and butter into the bowl and beat it well.
5. Add eggs and vanilla and combine at high speed until fluffy.
6. Mix the salt, baking soda, and flour into the bowl.

7. Add flour mixture and milk to the egg mixture and stir well.
8. Then, fold it into the bananas. Place mixture into the pan.
9. Bake it for one hour and ten minutes.
10. When done, place it into the freezer for forty-five minutes.

To prepare the frosting:
1. Cream the cream cheese and butter into the bowl. Add lemon juice and lemon zest and combine well.
2. Add powdered sugar and stir well. Top frosting over the cake.

Nutrition:
Calories; 470kcal, carbohydrates; 70g, protein; 5g, fat; 19g

169. Grilled Fish Steaks

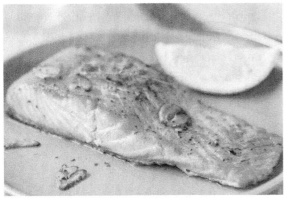

Preparation time: 10 minutes
Cooking time: 10 minutes
Additional time: 1 hour 10 minutes
Servings: 2
Ingredients:
- Garlic, one clove, minced
- Olive oil – six tbsp
- Dried basil – one tsp
- Salt – one tsp
- Ground black pepper – one tsp
- Lemon juice – one tbsp
- Fresh parsley – one tbsp, chopped
- Halibut fillets – six ounce

Directions:
1. Mix the parsley, lemon juice, pepper, salt, basil, olive oil, and garlic into the bowl.
2. Add halibut fillets into the glass dish and place marinade over it.
3. Place it into the refrigerator for one hour.

4. Oil the grate and preheat the grill on high heat.
5. Discard marinade and place halibut fillets onto the grill, and cook for five minutes per side.
6. When done, serve and enjoy!

Nutrition:
Calories; 554kcal, carbohydrates; 2.2g, protein; 36.3g, fat; 43.7g

170. Apple Pudding

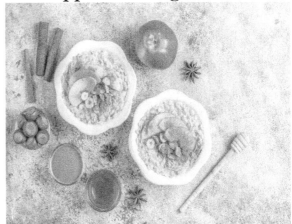

Preparation time: 10 minutes
Cooking time: 30 minutes
Servings: 6
Ingredients:
- Butter – half cup, melted
- White sugar – one cup
- All-purpose flour – one cup
- Baking powder – two tsp
- Salt – ¼ tsp
- Milk – one cup
- Apple – two cups, chopped and peeled
- Ground cinnamon – one tsp

Directions:
Preheat the oven to 375 degrees Fahrenheit.
Mix the milk, salt, baking powder, flour, sugar, and butter into the baking dish.

Mix the cinnamon and apples into the bowl and microwave it for two to five minutes. Place apple into the middle of the batter.

Place it into the oven and bake for a half-hour.

Serve and enjoy!

Nutrition:

Calories; 384kcal, carbohydrates; 57.5g, protein; 3.8g, fat; 16g

171. Lamb Chops

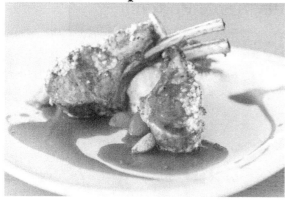

Preparation time: 30 minutes
Cooking time: 30 minutes
Servings: 2
Ingredients:

- Lamb chops – 2lb, cut ¾" thick, 4 pieces
- Kosher salt and Black pepper – for seasoning
- Garlic – one tbsp, minced
- Rosemary – two tsp, chopped
- Thyme – two tsp, chopped
- Parsley – half tsp, chopped
- Extra-virgin olive oil – ¼ cup

Directions:

1. Rub the lamb chops with pepper and salt.
2. Mix the two tbsp olive oil, parsley, thyme, rosemary, and garlic into the bowl.
3. Rub this paste on each side of the lamb chops and let marinate it for a half-hour.
4. Place two tbsp olive oil into the frying pan over medium-high flame.
5. Add lamb chops and cook for two to three minutes.
6. Flip and cook for three to four minutes more.
7. Let cool it for ten minutes.
8. Serve and enjoy!

Nutrition:

Calories; 465kcal, carbohydrates; 12g, protein; 14g, fat; 38g

172. Eggplant Croquettes

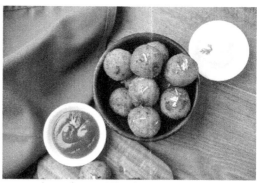

Preparation time: 15 minutes
Cooking time: 20 minutes
Servings: 6
Ingredients:

- Eggplants – two, peeled and cubed
- Cheddar cheese – one cup, shredded
- Italian seasoned bread crumbs – one cup
- Eggs – two, beaten
- Dried parsley – two tbsp
- Onion – two tbsp, chopped
- Garlic – one clove, minced
- Vegetable oil – one cup, for frying
- Salt – one tsp
- Ground black pepper – half tsp

Directions:

1. Microwave the eggplant over medium-high heat for three minutes.
2. Flip and cook for two minutes more.
3. If eggplant did not tender, cook for two minutes more.
4. Then, drain it and mash the eggplants.
5. Mix the salt, garlic, onion, parsley, eggs, cheese, breadcrumbs, and mashed eggplant.
6. Make the patties from the eggplant mixture.
7. Add oil into the skillet and heat it. Place eggplant patties into the skillet and fry until golden brown for five minutes.
8. Serve and enjoy!

Nutrition:

Calories; 266kcal, carbohydrates; 23.6g, protein; 12g, fat; 14.4g

173. Cucumber Egg Salad

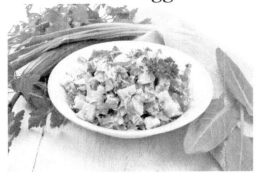

Preparation time: 10 minutes
Cooking time: 15 minutes
Servings: 4
Ingredients:

- Eggs – four
- Cucumbers – four, seedless
- Dill pickles – four
- Mayonnaise – three tbsp

Directions:

1. Add eggs into the saucepan and cover it with cold water. Let boil it.
2. Remove from the flame. Let stand eggs in hot water for ten to twelve minutes.
3. Remove from the hot water and cool it.
4. Peel eggs and chop them. Add it into the salad bowl.
5. Cube and pickled the cucumber and add to the eggs.
6. Add mayonnaise and combine it well.
7. Place it into the fridge until chill.

Nutrition:

Calories; 176kcal, carbohydrates; 8g, protein; 7.6g, fat; 13.4g

Chapter 12. Lunch high fiber

174. High-Fiber Dumplings

Preparation Time: 10 minutes
Cooking Time: 10 minutes
Servings: 8
Ingredients:

- 200 g cream quark
- 60 g psyllium husks
- 10 g bamboo fibers
- 1 bowl Vegetable broth
- 2 eggs

Directions:

1. Take a bowl and add the psyllium husks along with the bamboo fibers. Mix well with a spoon.
2. Put the eggs in the same bowl, add the cream curd and vegetable stock. Knead well, it's best done by hand. Alternatively, the kneading hooks of the mixer can be used.
3. Set a large saucepan with water and bring to a boil on the stove. In the meantime, moisten your hands with water and roll the dough into 12 balls.
4. Put the balls in the hot water and cook for 10 minutes, then serve. High-fiber vegetables like beans and matching sauces also taste great.

Nutrition:
Calories: 75
Carbs: 0.1 g
Protein: 13.4 g
Fat: 1.7 g
Sugar: 0 g
Sodium: 253 mg

175. Pizza Made with Bamboo Fibers

Preparation Time: 10 minutes
Cooking Time: 20 minutes
Servings: 4
Ingredients:

- 2 eggs
- 60 g bamboo fibers
- 80 g sour cream
- 40 g olive oil
- 150 g grated Gouda cheese
- Salt and pepper

Directions:

1. First, preheat the oven to 180ºC and cover a baking sheet with baking paper.
2. Take a bowl and beat in the eggs. Whisk briefly with a fork, then add the remaining ingredients and knead everything well. This is best done by hand, but you can also work with the dough hook on the mixer.
3. Finally, flavor with salt and pepper to taste, then place the dough on the baking tray and roll out evenly. If necessary, flour the dough with a little bamboo fiber so that the dough does not stick to the rolling pin.
4. Bake the tray for 10 minutes on the lower rack. The pizza base can now be topped with delicious low-carb foods, depending on your taste. Then bake for another 10 minutes on the lower rack and then enjoy hot.

Nutrition:
Calories: 599
Fat: 19 g
Carbs: 9 g
Sugar: 4 g
Fiber: 2 g
Protein: 97 g
Sodium: 520 mg

176. Vegetarian Hamburgers

Preparation Time: 10 minutes
Cooking Time: 30 minutes
Servings: 4
Ingredients:

- 90 g protein flour
- 120 ml egg white
- 100 g carrots, grated
- 2 tablespoons coconut oil
- 100 g low-fat quark
- 2 eggs
- 6 g baking powder
- 20 g gold linseed (alternatively other nuts and grains)
- Preferred spices (Worcester sauce, soy sauce, salt or chili)
- Preferred topping (tomatoes, cucumbers, radishes, ...)

Directions:

1. First, preheat the oven to 180°C and line 6-7 muffin tins with paper cases.
2. Take a bowl, add 50 g of flour along with the egg white and carrots, and then stir well. Divide the dough into 6-7 parts and shape a meatball from each one.
3. Now, put 2 tablespoons of coconut oil in a non-stick pan and heat over medium heat until it has melted. Put the meatballs in the hot pan and fry vigorously on both sides.
4. Take a separate bowl, add the remaining flour along with the low-fat quark, eggs, baking powder and gold linseed.
5. Mix well, then pour into the prepared muffin cups. Bake in the oven for 25 minutes, let the finished rolls cool down well. Finally, cut the rolls in half with a sharp knife, top with a meatball of your choice and season. Then, skewer the finished burger with a toothpick and enjoy.

Nutrition:
Calories: 178
Fat: 4 g
Carbs: 7 g
Fiber: 2 g
Protein: 27 g

177. Pork Steaks with Avocado
Preparation Time: 10 minutes
Cooking Time: 30 minutes
Servings: 8
Ingredients:
For the salsa:
- 6 limes
- 3 tablespoons fruity olive oil
- 1 ½ dried chili pepper
- Salt and freshly ground pepper
- 2 mangoes (ripe, but still firm)
- 2 shallots
- 2 avocados
- A bunch of coriander

For the steaks:
- 4 pork neck steaks (approximately 150 g each)
- 1 teaspoon ground anise
- 1 teaspoon ground cumin
- Salt
- freshly ground pepper
- 2 tablespoons clarified butter

Directions:
For the salsa:
1. Halve the limes and squeeze them thoroughly, measure out 10 tablespoons of lime juice. Place in a small bowl.
2. Add olive oil and stir well with a whisker. Crumble the chili pepper and mix into the dressing together with salt and pepper.
3. Now, peel the mangoes with a vegetable peeler, remove the stone and dice the pulp. Finely chop the shallots with a sharp knife.
4. Take a separate bowl, add the mangoes and shallots; stir well.
5. Remove the stone and skin from the avocados, dice the meat and then fill the mango mixture. Immediately, pour the dressing over it so that the avocado doesn't tarnish. Mix gently.
6. Finally, wash the coriander thoroughly under running water and dry it carefully. Remove the tender leaves and also add to the salsa. Mix again.

For the steaks:
7. Preheat the oven to 60°C. Rinse the steaks under running water and dry them carefully with a little kitchen roll. Sprinkle the anise, cumin, salt and pepper over them. Place the clarified butter in a pan and heat over medium heat until melted. Set the steaks in the hot pan and fry briefly while turning for 3 minutes.
8. Put the steaks on a piece of aluminum foil and seal it tightly around the steak. Place in the oven and let rest briefly for 3 minutes.
9. Arrange on a plate with the meat juice and salsa. Enjoy immediately!

Nutrition:
Calories: 303
Fat: 14 g
Carbs: 15 g
Sugar: 10 g
Fiber: 2 g
Protein: 30 g
Sodium: 387 mg

178. Chicken with Asparagus Salad
Preparation Time: 10 minutes

Cooking Time: 30 minutes
Servings: 4
Ingredients:

- 800 g green asparagus
- 1/2 bunch spring onions
- 3 tablespoons white wine vinegar
- Salt
- Pepper
- 1 teaspoon mustard
- 1/2 teaspoon honey
- 8 tablespoons olive oil
- 4 chicken breast fillets (approximately 200 g each)
- 250 g sliced breakfast bacon
- 2 tablespoons clarified butter
- Basil leaves for garnishing

Directions:

1. First, preheat the oven to 180°C and place baking paper on a baking sheet.
2. Take the asparagus and peel only the bottom stick.
3. Remove the woody ends, then wash thoroughly. Halve the asparagus lengthways and cut so that oblique pieces are created. Now, wash the spring onions and cut them into large pieces.
4. Take a bowl, pour the white wine vinegar into it. Also, attach 2 tablespoons of water along with mustard, honey, salt and pepper. Stir well.
5. Finally, slowly add 6 tablespoons of olive oil, spoon by spoon. Stir.
6. Take the meat, rinse under running water and dry with a little kitchen roll, then season with salt and pepper on both sides.
7. Take the bacon slices and wrap the meat in them.
8. Put the clarified butter in a non-stick pan and heat over medium fire until the fat has melted. Set the chicken breasts in the hot pan, first placing them to the point where the ends of the bacon slice meet. Turn after 2 minutes and fry again briefly for 2 minutes.
9. Remove from the pan and place on the tray so that the meat can cook in the oven for another 15 minutes.

   In the meantime, set the remaining olive oil in a pan and heat over medium fire. Put the vegetables in the hot oil and fry briefly. Meanwhile, salt and pepper. After 4 minutes, take the vegetables out of the pan and add them to the vinegar mixture, mix well.

   Finally, arrange the meat with the asparagus salad on a plate and enjoy immediately.

179. Hot Pepper and Lamb Salmon

Preparation Time: 10 minutes
Cooking Time: 20 minutes
Servings: 6
Ingredients:
For the Meat:

- 700 g lamb salmon
- 2 garlic cloves
- 1/2 bunch mint
- 2 sprigs rosemary
- 1/2 bunch oregano
- 10 peppercorns
- 4 tablespoons olive oil
- Salt
- Pepper

For the Peperonat:

- 1 small zucchini
- 2 red peppers
- 2 yellow peppers
- 1 onion
- 3 garlic cloves
- 3 tomatoes
- 1 chili pepper
- 3 tablespoon small capers
- 2 tablespoons olive oil
- Salt
- Pepper
- 2 tablespoons chopped parsley

Directions:
For the Meat:

1. First, rinse the meat under running water and dry it with a little kitchen roll, then carefully remove the tendons and fat. Peel and cut the garlic to make fine slices.
2. Wash the rosemary, oregano and mint, pat dry carefully. Then, chop the leaves and needles (not too fine). Put the peppercorns in the mortar and press lightly. Take a bowl, add the herbs and peppercorns.

3. Attach 2 tablespoons of olive oil and stir well, then rub the meat with the mixture. Finally, wrap it in foil and refrigerate for 4 hours.
4. Preheat the oven to 70ºC, placing a baking dish in it that will be used for the meat later.
5. Now, take the meat and remove the marinade with the back of a knife, then season with salt and pepper. Set the remaining oil in a pan and heat over medium fire.
6. Place the meat in the hot oil and fry briefly while turning for 2 minutes. Put it in the pan into the oven and cook for another 40 minutes.
7. For the Peperonata:
8. Wash the zucchini thoroughly and dice with the skin. Halve and core the peppers, wash them too. Cut so that narrow strips are created. First, peel the onion and garlic then process into fine cubes.
9. Score the tomatoes, pour hot water, at that time peel them and remove the seeds. Cut the pulp into small pieces. Alternatively, canned tomatoes can also be used here. Halve and core the chili pepper, wash it well and cut into small pieces. Finally, rinse the capers in a sieve and let them drain.
10. Now, pour olive oil over the pan and heat over medium fire. Put the onion in the hot oil and fry briefly, then add the peppers, zucchini, garlic and chili. Cook for 5 minutes, stirring evenly. Attach tomatoes and season with salt and pepper.
    a. Let everything fry for 10 minutes, stir in the capers and cook for another 5 minutes.

Nutrition:
Calories: 599
Fat: 19 g
Carbs: 9 g
Sugar: 4 g
Fiber: 2 g
Protein: 97 g
Sodium: 520 mg

180. Pork rolls à la Ratatouille

Preparation Time: 10 minutes
Cooking Time: 30 minutes
Servings: 8
Ingredients:

For the Ratatouille:
- 2 yellow peppers
- 2 red peppers
- 2 small zucchini
- 2 red onions
- 3 garlic cloves
- 250 g cherry tomatoes
- A bunch of thyme
- 3 tablespoons olive oil
- Salt
- Freshly ground pepper
- 250 ml vegetable stock
- 3 tablespoons tomato paste

For the Pork Rolls:
- 2 bunches basil
- 30 g Parmesan cheese
- 30 g pine nuts
- 5 tablespoons olive oil
- Salt
- Freshly ground pepper
- 75 g sun-dried tomatoes in oil
- 8 small pork schnitzel (approximately 75 g each)

Directions:
For the Ratatouille:
1. First, preheat the oven to 180ºC.
2. Halve and core the peppers, wash thoroughly and cut so that narrow strips are formed.
3. Wash the zucchini as well, then cut into cubes with the skin on. First, peel the onion and garlic then cut into strips. Clean the tomatoes thoroughly, cut them in half.
4. Rinse the thyme under running water and pat dry carefully, remove the leaves. Take a bowl, add the vegetables with the thyme and mix well.
5. Flavor with salt, pepper and olive oil; mix again. Take the frying pan from the oven and distribute the vegetable mixture in it. Bake for 20 minutes.
6. For the Pork Rolls:
7. Now, rinse the basil with water and shake dry, pluck the leaves and chop finely. Coarsely or finely grate the Parmesan with the grater to taste.
8. Take a small pan, add the pine nuts and briefly toast them without adding any

further fat, then put them in the blender. Also, add half of the chopped basil along with the Parmesan and 3 tablespoons of olive oil. Puree everything into a pesto, then season with salt and pepper.

9. Wash the tomatoes and cut them to make strips. Clean the pork as well, dry it with a little kitchen roll and then plate with a meat tenderizer or a saucepan. Sprinkle with salt and pepper, spread some pesto on top.

10. Spread the sun-dried tomatoes and the remaining basil on top, roll into roulades and set. Add the remaining oil to a pan and heat over medium fire, place the rolls in the hot oil and fry on all sides for 5 minutes.

    a. Take a small bowl, add the vegetable stock and tomato paste. Stir.

    b. Add the cherry tomatoes and the mixture to the cooked vegetables in the oven. Put the meat on it and bake for another 15 minutes. Enjoy served on a plate with the remaining pesto.

Nutrition:
Calories: 280
Fat: 16
Carbs: 5 g
Sugar: 1 g
Fiber: 0 g
Protein: 29 g

181. Pepper Fillet with Leek

Preparation Time: 10 minutes
Cooking Time: 30 minutes
Servings: 8
Ingredients:
For the Vegetables:

- 50 g sun-dried tomatoes
- 100 g pine nuts
- 4 large leeks
- 2 tablespoon raisins
- 2 cups Peppercorns
- 2 tablespoons olive oil
- Salt
- Freshly ground pepper

For the Meat:

- 2 tablespoons black pepper
- 4 tablespoons sesame seeds

- 1 teaspoon salt
- 4 sprigs rosemary
- 4 beef fillet steaks (approximately 180 g each)
- 4 tablespoons sunflower oil

Directions:

1. Place the tomatoes in a heat-resistant bowl and pour boiling water over them. Let stand for 10 minutes, then take out the tomatoes and chop with a sharp knife.

2. Now, put the pine nuts in a small pan and briefly toast them without adding any further fat, stirring well. Set aside and wash the leek thoroughly and cut so that rings are formed. Rinse the raisins under cold running water.

3. Take a non-stick pan and pour in olive oil. Heat on high and add the leek. Saute briefly, add tomatoes and raisins over low heat and stir well. Cook for 10 minutes, season with salt and pepper. Add the pine nuts then carefully stir in.

4. At the same time, put the peppercorns in the mortar and coarsely crush them, stir in a small bowl with salt and sesame seeds.

5. Rinse off the rosemary and steaks then dry them with a little paper towel. Place the steaks with the edges in the pepper mixture so that the spices stick to the edges.

6. Now, heat oil in a non-stick pan on a high level and sear the meat on both sides for 3 minutes. Immediately, wrap in a piece of aluminum foil, covering a sprig of rosemary with it.

7. After resting for 5 minutes, remove the steaks and arrange on a plate with the leek vegetables. Garnish with meat juice and enjoy instantly.

Nutrition:
Calories: 504
Fat: 39 g
Carbs: 10 g
Sugar: 1 g
Fiber: 2 g
Protein: 28 g
Sodium: 755 mg

182. Lamb Chops with Beans

Preparation Time: 10 minutes

Cooking Time: 50 minutes
Servings: 8
Ingredients:
- 1 kg lamb chops
- 2 lemons juice
- Salt
- Pepper
- 150 ml olive oil (approximately)
- 6 garlic cloves
- 6 sprigs rosemary
- 6 sprigs thyme
- 2 onions
- 12 cocktail tomatoes
- 300 g green beans
- 2 shallots
- 70 g bacon
- 2 teaspoons butter
- Savory to taste

Directions:
1. First, rinse the lamb chops briefly under running water and carefully dry them with a little kitchen roll. Pour the lemon juice into a small bowl, add 100 ml of olive oil, salt and pepper; stir well. Take the garlic and remove the peel. Cut so that thin slices are formed, also add to the lemon marinade.
2. Now, put the marinade together with the chops in a freezer bag, squeeze out the air and seal.
3. Set aside for at least 2 hours and let it soak in.
4. Preheat the oven to 180°C. Rinse the rosemary, thyme and pat dry. Take a baking dish and grease it with olive oil. Spread the herb sprigs in it.
5. Add the onions and cut into 4 parts, place them in the mold as well. Wash the tomatoes thoroughly and cut in half depending on the size, then add to the onions.
6. Set the meat out of the marinade and place it on top of the vegetables. Spread the soak and a little olive oil on top. Bake on the middle rack for 40 minutes.
7. In the meantime, take the beans and cut the ends, then wash. Set the water to a boil in a saucepan, season with salt and add the beans. Cook for 8 minutes. Meanwhile, take the shallots and remove the skin, cut into small cubes. Finely dice the bacon as well.
8. Put the butter in a pan and heat over medium fire until it has melted.
9. Place the shallots and bacon in the hot oil and fry until everything takes on a brown color.
10. Add the beans with a little savory, stir well.
11. Salt and pepper, then serve with the lamb and the bed of vegetables. Enjoy hot.

Nutrition:
Calories: 413
Fat: 20 g
Carbs: 7 g
Sugar: 1 g
Fiber: 1 g
Protein: 50 g
Sodium: 358 mg

183. Fillet of Beef on Spring Vegetables

Preparation Time: 10 minutes
Cooking Time: 30 minutes
Servings: 8
Ingredients:
- 500 g green asparagus
- 2 bulbs kohlrabi
- 1 bunch flat-leaf parsley
- 1 bunch tarragon
- Salt
- Pepper
- 4 beef fillet steaks (approximately 150 g each)
- 4 tablespoons olive oil
- 300 ml cream

Directions:
1. Wash the asparagus, peel only the bottom stick with the vegetable peeler. Divide off the woody ends, then cut the asparagus in half. Now, peel the kohlrabi with the knife, cut so that narrow sticks are formed.
2. Rinse the herbs under running water, dry them carefully and remove the leaves. Finely chop with a sharp knife. Take a bowl, pour in 2/3 of the herbs, set aside the rest for now.
3. After that, add the vegetables to the herbs in the bowl, season with salt and pepper and mix well. Put the mixture in a roasting tube (must be closed on one side).

4. Take a large saucepan, pour water up to 1/3 full. Set on the stove and bring to a boil.

5. In the meantime, rinse the steaks with water and dry them carefully with a little kitchen roll.

6. Season with salt and pepper on both sides. Put the oil in a pan and heat over medium fire.

7. Set the meat in the hot oil and fry briefly on all sides for 3 minutes. Place it on the vegetables in the roasting tube.

8. Pour the oil out of the pan and add in the cream. Bring to the boil briefly so that the roasting loosens, then pour over the meat in the roasting tube.

9. Now, close the hose and add it to the boiling water. Cook gently over low heat and cover for 12 minutes.

10. Finally, arrange the meat with the bed of vegetables on a plate and garnish with the remaining herbs.

Nutrition:
Calories: 209
Fat: 10 g
Carbs: 21 g
Sugar: 13 g
Fiber: 8 g
Protein: 11 g
Sodium: 644 mg

184. Bolognese with Zucchini Noodles

Preparation Time: 10 minutes
Cooking Time: 50 minutes
Servings: 4-8
Ingredients:
- 4 zucchini (approximately 200 g each)
- Salt
- 1 onion
- 3 garlic cloves
- 2 tablespoons coconut oil
- 4 tablespoons tomato paste
- 3 tablespoons balsamic vinegar
- 600 g chunky tomatoes (canned)
- 4 sprigs rosemary
- 1 handful basil leaves
- 1/2tbsp. Dried oregano
- 1/4tsp. Dried thyme

- Freshly ground black pepper
- 600 g mixed minced meat
- 2 tablespoons olive oil

Directions:
1. First, wash the zucchini and cut them into thin, narrow slices.

2. For preparing the Bolognese, peel the onion and garlic; cut into fine cubes. Set the oil in a saucepan and heat over medium fire. Put the onion in the hot oil and fry until it becomes translucent.

3. Stir well and fry briefly before adding the tomato paste. Cook them together again, pour in the balsamic vinegar until the bottom can no longer be seen. Bring to a boil, add the tomatoes.

4. Wash the rosemary, and basil then dry them carefully. Pluck the needles and leaves, chop and add to the Bolognese. Season with the remaining herbs to taste.

5. Reduce the heat and simmer gently for 30 minutes before stirring in the minced meat. Cook for another 15 minutes, then cook over high heat for 5 minutes.

6. At the same time, attach olive oil to the zucchini noodles and mix well.

7. Put the oiled zucchini in a pan and cook only briefly over medium heat without becoming too soft.

8. Arrange with the Bolognese on a plate and enjoy hot.

Nutrition:
Calories: 75
Carbs: 0.1 g
Protein: 13.4 g
Fat: 1.7 g
Sugar: 0 g
Sodium: 253 mg

185. Chicken with Chickpeas

Preparation Time: 10 minutes
Cooking Time: 30 minutes
Servings: 4
Ingredients:
- 12 sun-dried tomatoes in oil
- 2 garlic cloves
- 2 zucchini
- 500 g chickpeas (canned, drained weight)
- 4 tablespoons olive oil

- 100 ml poultry stock
- 2 bags saffron threads
- Salt
- Freshly ground black pepper
- 1/4 teaspoon ground coriander
- 4 chicken breasts (approximately 200 g each)
- 1 tbsp. Ras el Hanout

Directions:
1. First, get the sun-dried tomatoes out of the oil and dry them with a little kitchen roll, then cut them so that narrow strips are formed.
2. Take the garlic, remove the skin and cut into slices.
3. Wash the zucchini and cut into cubes with the skin on.
4. Rinse the chickpeas in a colander and drain well.
5. Set a saucepan, add 2 tablespoons of olive oil. Warmth on medium heat, add the tomatoes with garlic to the hot oil. Fry briefly for 1 minute.
6. Place the zucchini with chickpeas, stir well and fry briefly together before deglazing with the broth. Add saffron threads, coriander, salt and pepper. Bring to a boil.
7. Set the heat, cover the saucepan and let the vegetables simmer for 5 minutes.
8. In the meantime, rinse the meat under running water and dry it with a little kitchen roll. Set the remaining oil in a pan and heat over medium fire.
9. For now, sprinkle the meat on both sides with salt, pepper and Ras el Hanout, then add to the hot oil and fry for 7 minutes, turning.
10. Serve the meat with the vegetables on a large plate and enjoy hot.

Nutrition:
Calories: 329
Fat: 17 g
Carbs: 9 g
Sugar: 3 g
Fiber: 5 g
Protein: 37 g
Sodium: 430 mg

186. Ham with Chicory

Preparation Time: 10 minutes

Cooking Time: 30 minutes
Servings: 4-8
Ingredients:
- 4 sprigs chicory (approximately 200 g each)
- 150 g Emmental cheese
- 8 sage leaves
- 40 g butter
- 3 tablespoons orange juice
- Salt
- Pepper
- 8 slices Black Forest ham

Directions:
1. First, preheat the oven to 200ºC.
2. Wash and clean the chicory and cut it lengthways in half. Remove the stalk with a knife.
3. Shred the cheese coarsely or finely with a grater to taste.
4. Rinse the sage leaves under running water and gently shake dry.
5. Put the butter in a pan and heat over medium fire. Extinguish with orange juice and so froth the butter. Add the sage.
6. Place the chicory with the cut side in the hot oil. Reduce the heat and fry for 5 minutes.
7. Remove the chicory, cover with a sage leaf and sprinkle with salt and pepper.
8. Chop the ham and put it on the baking dish. Sprinkle with cheese and drizzle with liquid orange and butter. Bake in the oven for 20 minutes, then serve hot.

Nutrition:
Calories: 75
Carbs: 0.1 g
Protein: 13.4 g
Fat: 1.7 g
Sugar: 0 g
Sodium: 253 mg

187. Pork medallions with asparagus and coconut curry

Preparation Time: 10 minutes
Cooking Time: 30 minutes
Servings: 4-8
Ingredients:
- 1 kg white asparagus
- 500 g carrots
- 2 onions
- 1 red chili pepper

- 40 g butter
- 3-4 tablespoons curry powder
- 250 ml vegetable stock
- 400 ml coconut milk
- 2–3 tablespoons lime juice
- Salt
- Pepper
- 1 tablespoon chopped coriander
- 4 pork medallions (125 g each)
- 2-3 tablespoons oil

Directions:

1. First, peel the asparagus and remove the woody ends, wash well and cut into bite-sized pieces. Then, peel the carrots, wash and cut them into slices. Now, take the onions, remove the skin and cut them into cubes. Divide the chili in half, take out the seeds and carefully dice.
2. Put the butter in a pan and heat over medium fire until it has melted.
3. Put the onions and chili in the hot oil and saute until translucent. Add asparagus, carrots and fry everything for 5 minutes, stirring regularly.
4. Pour the curry over it and fry briefly before adding the broth. Set the heat, cover the saucepan and simmer for 15 minutes.
5. Add in the coconut milk and cook for 3 more minutes. Pour in lime juice, salt and pepper to taste. Sprinkle on 1/2 tablespoon of coriander; stir well.
6. Now, take the meat and season with salt and pepper on both sides. Put the oil in a pan and heat over medium fire.
7. Place the medallions in the hot oil and fry briefly on both sides for about 3-5minutes.
8. Arrange medallions with curry on a plate, garnish with coriander and serve hot.

Nutrition:

Calories: 432
Fat: 12 g
Carbs: 12 g
Sugar: 5 g
Fiber: 3 g
Protein: 57 g
Sodium: 566 mg

188. Lamb with Carrot and Brussels Sprouts Spaghetti

Preparation Time: 10 minutes
Cooking Time: 30 minutes
Servings: 4-8
Ingredients:

- 250 g Brussels sprouts
- 300 g carrots
- 5 tablespoons sesame oil
- 3 tablespoons soy sauce
- 1 lime juice
- A pinch of sugar
- Salt
- 600 g loosened saddle of lamb
- Pepper
- 2 tablespoons butter
- 2 tablespoons sesame seeds

Directions:

1. First, preheat the oven to 100°C.
2. Take the Brussels sprouts, wash and clean. Then, cut them into strips.
3. For preparing the marinade, place 3 tablespoons of sesame oil together with soy sauce, sugar, salt and lime juice in a bowl; merge well.
4. Put the vegetable spaghetti in the marinade and let it steep for a moment.
5. In the meantime, flavor the lamb with salt and pepper. Pour the remaining oil into a coated pan and heat on high.
6. Set the meat in the hot oil and sear it on all sides, then put it in the oven and let it cook gently for 10 minutes.
7. After that, melt the butter in the same pan and fry the marinated vegetables for about 3-4 minutes. Arrange on a plate with the sliced lamb and garnish with sesame seeds.

Nutrition:

Calories: 270
Fat: 11 g
Carbs: 4 g
Sugar: 1 g
Fiber: 1 g
Protein: 39 g
Sodium: 664 mg

189. Cabbage Wrap

Preparation Time: 10 minutes

Cooking Time: 30 minutes
Servings: 4-8
Ingredients:

- 1 head white cabbage
- Salt
- 100 ml milk
- 1 roll (from the day before)
- 350 g mixed minced meat
- 1 egg freshly ground pepper
- 2 tablespoons clarified butter
- 250 ml meat stock
- 1 tablespoon flour
- 4 tablespoons cream

Directions:

1. First, separate the large outer leaves (12-16 pieces) from the cabbage and cut out the strong leaf veins with a knife. Set a saucepan with water and bring to a boil. Salt well and add the large cabbage leaves with the rest of the cabbage. Cook everything for 5-10 minutes.
2. Heat the milk in a saucepan. Put the roll on it and soak for a few minutes.
3. Squeeze out the bun and place in a bowl. Also add the minced meat, egg, pepper and salt. Mix everything well until a batter is formed.
4. Cut the cooked cabbage (not the large leaves) and add to the dough, mix again.
5. Take 3-4 cabbage leaves and stack them on top of each other. Spread some batter on top, then roll the leaves and fix with toothpicks, roulade needles, or kitchen twine.
6. Put the clarified butter in a pan and heat over medium fire until it melts. Then, place the cabbage rolls in the hot oil and fry them lightly brown.
7. Extinguish with the broth, cover the pan and simmer the cabbage rolls over low heat for 25 minutes. Take out the cabbage rolls and briefly keep them warm.
8. Now, stir in the flour in a little cream and add everything to the sauce. Bring to a boil briefly.
9. Arrange on plates with the cabbage rolls.
   Nutrition:

Calories: 329
Fat: 17 g
Carbs: 9 g
Sugar: 3 g
Fiber: 5 g
Protein: 37 g

190. Veal with Asparagus
Preparation Time: 10 minutes
Cooking Time: 30 minutes
Servings: 4-8
Ingredients:

- 800 g green asparagus
- Salt
- 3-4 tablespoons rapeseed oil
- A pinch of sugar
- Pepper
- 1/2 fresh lemon zest, grated
- Oil for frying
- 8 slices veal from the back (60 g each)
- 8 slices Parma ham
- 8 sage leaves
- 125 ml white wine
- 1 tablespoon butter

Directions:

1. First, peel the lower part of the sticks with a vegetable peeler, then remove the woody ends. Wash the asparagus thoroughly.
2. At the same time, fill a saucepan with water and bring it to a boil. Salt well, add the asparagus, and cook for 8 minutes, they must not become too soft. Drain them and rinse directly with ice water.
3. Place the asparagus on a piece of kitchen roll to dry, then put them in a baking dish.
4. Take a small bowl and add the oil, salt, pepper, sugar 0and lemon zest. Mix everything well and pour over the asparagus stalks. Let sit in the marinade for 25 minutes.
5. Put the oil in a pan and heat over medium fire. Detach the asparagus from the marinade and place them in the hot oil. Fry while turning.
6. Now, pepper the meat and cover it with Parma ham and a sage leaf. Secure everything with a toothpick.
7. Put the oil in a pan, heat it and place the meat in it. Fry briefly on medium heat and turning for 3 minutes.
8. Serve with the asparagus on a plate. Extinguish the now-empty pan with white

wine so that the roasting residue dissolves, then stir in the butter and briefly bring to a boil.

9. Pour the sauce over the asparagus and meat. Enjoy hot.

Nutrition:

Calories: 599

Fat: 19 g

Carbs: 9 g

Sugar: 4 g

Fiber: 2 g

Protein: 97 g

Sodium: 520 mg

191. Salmon with Sesame Seeds and Mushrooms

Preparation Time: 10 minutes

Cooking Time: 30 minutes

Servings: 4-8

Ingredients:

- 500 g salmon fillet
- 4 tablespoons fish sauce
- 200 g mushrooms
- 400 g fresh spinach leaves
- 2 tablespoons vegetable oil
- 2 tablespoons sesame oil
- 1 tablespoon sesame seeds
- 1 teaspoon sambal oelek

Directions:

1. First, take the salmon, rinse under running water, dry with a little kitchen roll, and then cut so that strips are formed. Take a bowl, pour in the fish sauce. Soak the salmon in the sauce for 10 minutes.
2. In the meantime, it is best to carefully clean the mushrooms with a brush, cut them to make slices. Rinse and dry the spinach under the tap.
3. Now, take a wok, add the vegetable and sesame oil. Heat on high, add the mushrooms to the hot oil, and fry briefly. Put the spinach in the wok and fry until it collapses.
4. Now, move the vegetables away from the center to the edge of the wok and reduce the heat.
5. Place the salmon on the resulting surface and fry gently while turning.

6. Arrange it with the vegetables on a plate, carefully refine with sambal oelek to taste.

Nutrition:

Calories: 599

Fat: 19 g

Carbs: 9 g

Sugar: 4 g

Fiber: 2 g

Protein: 97 g

Sodium: 520 mg

192. Stuffed Trout with Mushrooms

Preparation Time: 10 minutes

Cooking Time: 30 minutes

Servings: 4-8

Ingredients:

- 4 ready-to-cook trout
- 1 lemon juice
- Salt
- Pepper
- 1/2 bunch dill
- 500 g mushrooms
- 2 tablespoons butter
- 2 tablespoons freshly chopped parsley
- 3 tablespoons chopped almonds
- 4 tablespoons oil

Directions:

1. First, preheat the oven to 220°C.
2. Take the lemon juice and use it to drizzle the trout inside and out. Wash the dill, shake dry and chop.
3. Salt and pepper the trout and refine each with 1 tablespoon of dill. It is best to carefully clean the mushrooms with a brush and cut them into slices.
4. Then, put them in a bowl. Also add the butter, almonds and parsley. Stir everything well.
5. Now, distribute the filling over the trout's abdominal cavities. Fix the abdomen with wooden skewers, wrap the trout well in aluminum foil coated with oil. Let it cook in the oven for 20 minutes.
6. Finally, put the fish on a plate and enjoy hot.

Nutrition:

Calories: 413

Fat: 20 g

Carbs: 7 g
Sugar: 1 g
Fiber: 1 g
Protein: 50 g
Sodium: 358 mg

Sugar: 13 g
Fiber: 8 g
Protein: 11 g
Sodium: 644 mg

193. Salmon with Basil and Avocado

Preparation Time: 10 minutes
Cooking Time: 30 minutes
Servings: 4-8
Ingredients:

- 1 avocado
- 1 teaspoon pickled capers
- 3 garlic cloves
- A handful of basil leaves
- 1 tablespoon fresh lemon zest
- 4 salmon fillets (approximately 200 g each)
- Coconut oil for greasing the tray

Directions:
1. Preheat the oven at 180ºC and use a brush to spread coconut oil on a baking sheet.
2. Divide the avocado in half, then remove the core and skin.
3. Mash the pulp with a fork in a small bowl.
4. Put the capers in a colander and drain, chop finely.
5. Peel the garlic cloves and mash them with a press. Alternatively, chop them very finely with a sharp knife.
6. Then, wash the basil and shake it dry, pluck the leaves off and chop them too.
7. Attach everything to the avocado in the bowl, refine with lemon zest and mix well.
8. Wash the salmon, dry with a little kitchen roll, and place on the baking sheet. It is best to spread the avocado mixture over the fish with a spoon.
9. Put the tray in the oven and bake briefly for 10 minutes. Switch on the grill function and bake for another 4 minutes until the avocado takes on a light brown color.
10. Set the salmon fillets on a plate and enjoy hot.

Nutrition:
Calories: 209
Fat: 10 g
Carbs: 21 g

194. Leek Quiche with Olives

Preparation Time: 10 minutes
Cooking Time: 30 minutes
Servings: 4-8
Ingredients:

- 140 g almonds
- 40 g walnuts
- 25 g coconut oil
- 1 teaspoon salt
- 1 leek
- 50 g spinach
- 2 sprigs rosemary
- 40 g fresh basil
- 30 g pine nuts
- 4 tablespoons extra-virgin olive oil
- 2 tablespoons lime juice
- 1/2 garlic clove
- 50 g pitted black olives
- 1 teaspoon red pepper berries

Directions:
1. First, coarsely grind the almonds and walnuts in a food processor or blender, then put them in a small bowl together with the coconut oil and 1/2 teaspoon of salt.
2. Merge thoroughly, pour the mixture into a cake springform pan. Press the dough with your fingers at the same time and distribute it in the mold so that a border of 4 cm high is created. Put it in the freezer for 15 minutes.
3. Now, wash the leek, spinach and herbs, then pat dry. Slice the leek and place it in a bowl.
4. Stir in the remaining salt and set aside to draw.
5. Meanwhile, put the basil, pine nuts, olive oil, and lime juice in a blender. Pulse until you have a creamy puree.
6. Alternatively, a large mixing vessel or a hand blender can also be used here.
7. Now, peel the garlic clove and chop half. Remove the needles from the rosemary and also finely chop them.

8. Cut the spinach into narrow strips and halve the olives.
9. Add everything to the leek in the bowl, and then add the basil puree. Mix well.
10. Distribute the mixture to the base of the springform pan, sprinkle the pepper berries over it. Finally, cut the quiche into pieces and enjoy.

Nutrition:
Calories: 270
Fat: 11 g
Carbs: 4 g
Sugar: 1 g
Fiber: 1 g
Protein: 39 g
Sodium: 664 mg

195. Fried Egg on Onions with Sage

Preparation Time: 10 minutes
Cooking Time: 30 minutes
Servings: 4-8
Ingredients:
- 275 g onions
- 1/2 bunch sage
- 3 tablespoons clarified butter
- 1 ½ tablespoon coconut flour
- Salt
- 1 teaspoon sweet paprika powder
- 8 eggs
- Freshly ground black pepper

Directions:
1. First, remove the skin from the onions, then cut into thin rings.
2. Rinse the sage under running water, pat dry and remove the leaves.
3. Now, put 1 ½ tablespoon of clarified butter in a pan and heat over medium fire until it has melted. Place the sage leaves in the hot oil and fry until they are crispy. Place on kitchen paper to drain.
4. Meanwhile, put the remaining clarified butter in the same pan and heat it, then place the onion rings in it.
5. Scatter the coconut flour on top and fry for 10 minutes, stirring at regular intervals. Sprinkle salt and paprika too.

6. Take the eggs and beat them one by one on the onions in the pan. Let the eggs sink to the bottom of the pan, if necessary use a wooden spoon to help.
7. Now, cover the pan and fry everything for 10 minutes until the eggs are completely set.
8. Arrange the fried eggs with the onions on flat plates, season with salt and pepper. Garnish with the roasted sage.

Nutrition:
Calories: 179
Fat: 13 g
Carbs: 6 g
Sugar: 3 g
Fiber: 1 g
Protein: 10 g
Sodium: 265 mg

196. Quinoa Mushroom Risotto

Preparation Time: 10 minutes
Cooking Time: 30 minutes
Servings: 4-8
Ingredients:
- 1 garlic clove
- 30 g hazelnuts
- Salt
- 1 fresh lemon zest, grated
- 2 shallots
- 650 g small mushrooms
- 1 bunch flat-leaf parsley
- 70 g quinoa
- 2 tablespoons olive oil
- Pepper
- 100 g baby spinach
- 30 g grated Parmesan cheese
- 20 g butter
- Red pepper to taste
- 500 ml hot water

Directions:
1. First, peel the garlic clove and put it in a blender. Also add the hazelnuts, lemon zest and a little salt; mix until everything is finely ground. Put aside.
2. Peel the shallots, then cut them into fine cubes. It is best to carefully clean the mushrooms with a brush, chop them so that thin slices are formed.

3. Rinse and dab the parsley under running water, remove the leaves and chop with a sharp knife.
4. Put the quinoa in a colander and wash well under the tap; drain thoroughly.
5. Pour olive oil into a non-stick pan and warmth over medium heat. Put the shallots in it and fry until they turn slightly brown.
6. Add the mushrooms to the shallots and fry them together until they turn brown. Attach the quinoa, but at the same time pour in the hot water. Season with salt and pepper, stir well.
7. Cook over low heat until all the water has boiled away. The quinoa should be soft.
8. Now, add the parsley, spinach, Parmesan and butter; stir thoroughly.
9. Salt and pepper again and set with garlic and the hazelnut mixture.
10. Arrange on a plate and serve garnished with red pepper if necessary.

Nutrition:
Calories: 166
Fat: 10 g
Carbs: 17 g
Sugar: 12 g
Fiber: 2 g
Protein: 7 g
Sodium: 892 mg

197. Vegetarian Lentil Stew

Preparation Time: 10 minutes
Cooking Time: 30 minutes
Servings: 4
Ingredients:
50 g carrots
- 30 g parsnip or parsley root
- 30 g celery
- 1 leek
- 1 yellow pepper
- 250 g red lentils
- 1 ½ teaspoon ground cumin
- 3 tablespoons balsamic vinegar
- 3 tablespoons walnut oil
- 2-3 tablespoons maple syrup
- Salt and pepper
- A pinch of cayenne pepper
- 1/2 bunch flat-leaf parsley

Directions:
1. Measure 1000 ml of water and pour into a saucepan. Warmth on high heat until boil.
2. In the meantime, cut the peppers in half, remove the seeds and wash them together with the leek. Peel the carrots, parsnips and celery.
3. Process everything into fine cubes, only use the white part of the leek.
4. Pour everything into the boiling water and bring to a boil. Then, add the lentils. Cook for 10 minutes, or until they are soft.
5. Ideally, most of the liquid has boiled away, if necessary drain. Season with cumin, balsamic vinegar, maple syrup, walnut oil, salt and pepper. Add the cayenne pepper to taste.
6. Turn off the stove and set the vegetarian lentils stew aside briefly to steep.
7. In the meantime, rinse the parsley under the tap, pat dry, pluck the leaves off and sprinkle them into the stew.
8. Arrange in deep plates and enjoy hot.

Nutrition:
Calories: 413
Fat: 20 g
Carbs: 7 g
Sugar: 1 g
Fiber: 1 g
Protein: 50 g
Sodium: 358 mg

198. Lemon Chicken Soup with Beans

Preparation Time: 10 minutes
Cooking Time: 50 minutes
Servings: 4
Ingredients:
- 1 onion
- 6 garlic cloves
- 600 g chicken breast
- 3 tablespoons olive oil
- l chicken broth
- 1 fresh lemon
- 250 g cooked white beans (canned)
- Salt
- Pepper

- 120 g Feta
- A bunch of chives

Directions:

1. First, peel the onion, then the garlic cloves. Divide the onion in half and cut it into thin slices.
2. Rinse the meat under running water and dry it with a little paper towel.
3. Put the olive oil in a large saucepan and heat over medium fire, add the onion and garlic to the hot oil.
4. Fry until everything is soft, deglaze with the chicken stock. Also, add the meat and bring to a boil.
5. In the meantime, wash and dry the lemon, then rub and peel it with a grater, alternatively, you can also use a zester. Add the lemon zest to the broth and cook everything for 40 minutes before adding the beans. Salt and pepper, then cook again for 10 minutes.
6. Now, remove the meat and tear it into small pieces on a plate or board with 2 forks. Put the chicken back into the soup, then crumble the Feta over the soup.
7. Finally, rinse the chives with water, dry and cut them so that small rolls are created. Sprinkle into the soup, stir well and immediately enjoy hot.

Nutrition:

Calories: 329
Fat: 17 g
Carbs: 9 g
Sugar: 3 g
Fiber: 5 g
Protein: 37 g
Sodium: 430 mg

Chapter 13. Dinner clear liquid

199. Homemade Beef Stock

Preparation Time: 10 minutes
Cooking Time: 2-12 hours
Servings: 6
Ingredients:

- 2 pounds beef bones (preferably with marrow)
- 5 celery stalks, chopped
- 4 carrots, chopped
- 1 white or Spanish onion, chopped
- 2 garlic cloves, crushed
- 2 bay leaves
- 1 teaspoon dried thyme
- 1 teaspoon dried sage
- 1 teaspoon black peppercorns
- Salt

Directions:

1. Preheat the oven to 425°F.
2. On a baking sheet, spread out the beef bones, celery, carrots, onion, garlic, and bay leaves. Sprinkle the thyme, sage, and peppercorns over the top.
3. Roast until the vegetables and bones have a rich brown color.
4. Transfer the roasted bones and vegetables to a large stockpot. Cover with water and slowly bring to a boil over high heat.
5. Set the heat to medium-low for at least 2 hours and up to 12 hours.
6. Pour the mixture through a fine-mesh strainer into a large bowl.
7. Taste and season with salt. Serve hot.

Nutrition:
Calories: 37
Fat: 1 g
Carbs: 3 g
Fiber: 0 g
Protein: 4 g
Sodium: 58 mg

200. Three-Ingredient Sugar-Free Gelatin

Preparation Time: 5 minutes
Cooking Time: 0 minutes
Servings: 6-8
Ingredients:

- 1/4 cup room temperature water
- 1/4 cup hot water
- 1 tablespoon gelatin
- 1 cup orange juice, unsweetened

Directions:

1. Combine your gelatin and room temperature water, stirring until fully dissolved.
2. Stir in hot water then leave to rest for about 2 minutes.
3. Add in the juice and stir until combined.
4. Transfer to serving size containers then place on a tray in the refrigerator to set for about 4 hours.
5. Enjoy!

Nutrition:
Calories: 17
Fat: 0 g
Carbs: 4 g
Fiber: 0 g
Protein: 0 g

201. Cranberry-Kombucha Jell-O

Preparation Time: 5 minutes
Cooking Time: 0 minutes
Servings: 6
Ingredients:

- 1/4 cup room temperature water
- 1/4 cup hot water
- 1 tablespoon gelatin
- 1 cup cranberry kombucha, unsweetened

Directions:

Combine your gelatin and room temperature water, stirring until fully dissolved.
Stir in hot water then leave to rest for about 2 minutes.
Add in the kombucha and stir until combined.
Transfer to serving size containers then place on a tray in the refrigerator to set for about 4 hours.
Enjoy!

Nutrition:
Calories: 13
Fat: 0 g
Carbs: 1 g
Fiber: 0 g
Protein: 0 g

202. Strawberry Gummies

Preparation Time: 5 minutes
Cooking Time: 5 minutes
Servings: 20-40 mini gummies
Ingredients:

- 1 cup strawberries, hulled and chopped
- 3/4 cup water
- 2 tablespoons gelatin

Directions:

1. Bring your water and berries to a boil on high heat. Detach from the heat as soon as the mixture begins to boil.
2. Transfer to the blender and pulse. Add in your gelatin then blend once more.
3. Pour the mixture into a silicone gummy mold.
4. Place on a tray in the refrigerator to set for about 4 hours.

Enjoy!
Nutrition:
Calories: 3
Fat: 0 g
Carbs: 0 g
Fiber: 0 g
Protein: 0 g

203. Fruity Jell-O Stars

Preparation Time: 15 minutes
Cooking Time: 5 minutes
Servings: 4
Ingredients:

- 1 tablespoon gelatin, powdered
- 3/4 cup boiling water
- 3 ½ cups fruit
- 1 tablespoon honey
- 1 teaspoon lemon juice

Directions:

1. Attach all your ingredients into a blender and pulse.
2. Add in the gelatin then blend once more.
3. Pour the mixture into a silicone gummy mold.
4. Place on a tray in the refrigerator to set for about 4 hours.
5. Enjoy!

Nutrition:
Calories: 2
Fat: 14 g

Carbs: 0 g
Fiber: 1 g
Protein: 0 g

204. Sugar-Free Cinnamon Jelly

Preparation Time: 5 minutes
Cooking Time: 0 minutes
Servings: 2
Ingredients:

- 1 cup hot cinnamon tea
- 1 cup room temperature water
- 2 teaspoons gelatin
- 1/3 cup sweetener

Directions:

1. Combine your gelatin and room temperature water, stirring until fully dissolved.
2. Stir in hot tea then leave to rest for about 2 minutes.
3. Add in the sweetener and stir until combined.
4. Transfer to serving size containers then place on a tray in the refrigerator to set for about 4 hours.
5. Enjoy!

Nutrition:
Calories: 35
Fat: 0 g
Carbs: 17 g
Fiber: 0 g
Protein: 0 g

205. Homey Clear Chicken Broth

Preparation Time: 10 minutes
Cooking Time: 2-12 hours
Servings: 6 cups
Ingredients:

- 2 pounds chicken neck
- 2 celery ribs with leaves, cut into chunks
- 2 medium carrots, cut into chunks
- 2 medium onions, quartered
- 2 bay leaves
- 2 quarts cold water
- Salt

Directions:

1. Transfer the bones and vegetables to your stockpot. Top with enough water to cover

then allow to come to a boil on high heat slowly.
2. Switch to low heat and simmer for at least 2 hours and up to 12 hours.
3. Set and pour the mixture through a fine-mesh strainer into a large bowl.
4. Taste and season with salt.
5. Serve hot.

Nutrition:
Calories: 245
Fat: 14 g
Carbs: 8 g
Fiber: 2 g
Protein: 21 g

206. Oxtail Bone Broth

Preparation Time: 15 minutes
Cooking Time: 12 hours
Servings: 8 cups
Ingredients:

- 2 pounds Oxtail
- 1 Onion, chopped in quarters
- 2 celery stalks, chopped in half
- 2 carrots, chopped in half
- 3 whole garlic cloves
- 2 bay leaves
- 1 tablespoon salt
- Filtered water (enough to cover bones)

Directions:
1. Transfer the bones and vegetables to your stockpot. Top with enough water to cover then allow to come to a boil on high heat slowly.
2. Switch to low heat and simmer for at least 2 hours and up to 12 hours.
3. Set and pour the mixture through a fine-mesh strainer into a large bowl.
4. Taste and season with salt.
5. Serve hot.

Nutrition:
Calories: 576
Fat: 48 g
Carbs: 48 g
Fiber: 0 g
Protein: 24 g

207. Chicken Bone Broth with Ginger and Lemon

Preparation Time: 10 minutes
Cooking Time: 90 minutes
Servings: 8
Ingredients:

- 3-4 pounds bones (from 1 chicken)
- 8 cups water
- 2 large carrots, cut into chunks
- 2 large stalks celery
- 1 large onion
- 3 fresh rosemary sprigs
- 3 fresh thyme sprigs
- 2 tablespoons apple cider vinegar
- 1 teaspoon kosher salt
- 1 (1/2 inches) piece fresh ginger, sliced (peeling not necessary)
- 1 large lemon, cut into quarters

Directions:
1. Put all the ingredients in your pot and allow to sit for 30 minutes.
2. Pressure cook and adjust the time to 90 minutes.
3. Set the broth using a fine-mesh strainer and transfer it into a storage container.
4. Can be refrigerated for 5 days or frozen for 6 months.

Nutrition:
Calories: 44 kcal
Fat: 1 g
Protein: 7 g
Sodium: 312 mg
Fiber: 0 g
Carbs: 0 g
Sugar: 0 g

208. Vegetable Stock

Preparation Time: 10 minutes
Cooking Time: 40 minutes
Servings: 8
Ingredients:
2 large carrots

- 1 large onion
- 2 large stalks celery
- 8 ounces white mushrooms
- 5 whole garlic cloves
- 2 cups parsley leaves

- 2 bay leaves
- 2 teaspoons whole black peppercorns
- 2 teaspoons kosher salt
- 10 cups water

Directions:
1. Place all the ingredients in your pot. Secure the lid.
2. Pressure cook and adjust the time to 40 minutes.
3. Set the broth using a fine-mesh strainer and transfer it into a storage container.

Nutrition:
Calories: 9
Fat: 0 g
Protein: 0 g
Sodium: 585 mg
Fiber: 0 g
Carbs: 2 g
Sugar: 1 g

209. Chicken Vegetable Soup
Preparation Time: 23 minutes
Cooking Time: 15 minutes
Servings: 8
Ingredients:
- 2 tablespoons avocado oil
- 1 small yellow onion, peeled and chopped
- 2 large carrots, peeled and chopped
- 2 large stalks celery, ends removed and sliced
- 3 garlic cloves, minced
- 1 teaspoon dried thyme
- 1 teaspoon salt
- 8 cups chicken stock
- 3 boneless, skinless, frozen chicken breasts

Directions:
1. Heat the oil for 1 minute. Add the onion, carrots, and celery and saute for 8 minutes.
2. Add the garlic, thyme, and salt then saute for another 30 seconds. Press the Cancel button.
3. Add the stock and frozen chicken breasts to the pot. Secure the lid.
4. Pressure cook and adjust the time to 6 minutes.
5. Allow cooling into bowls to serve.

Nutrition:
Calories: 209
Fat: 7 g
Protein: 21 g

Sodium: 687 mg
Fiber: 1 g
Carbs: 12 g
Sugar: 5 g

210. Carrot Ginger Soup
Preparation Time: 20 minutes
Cooking Time: 21 minutes
Servings: 4
Ingredients:
- 1 tablespoon avocado oil
- 1 large yellow onion, peeled and chopped
- 1 pound carrots, peeled and chopped
- 1 tablespoon fresh ginger, peeled and minced
- 1 ½ teaspoon salt
- 3 cups vegetable broth

Directions:
1. Add the oil to the inner pot, allowing it to heat for 1 minute.
2. Attach the onion, carrots, ginger, and salt then saute for 5 minutes. Press the Cancel button.
3. Add the broth and secure the lid. Adjust the time to 15 minutes.
4. Allow the soup to cool a few minutes and then transfer it to a large blender. Merge on high until smooth and then serve.

Nutrition:
Calories: 99
Fat: 4 g
Protein: 1 g
Sodium: 1,348 mg
Fiber: 4 g
Carbs: 16 g
Sugar: 7 g

211. Turkey Sweet Potato Hash
Preparation Time: 10 minutes
Cooking Time: 12 minutes
Servings: 4
Ingredients:
- 1 ½ tablespoon avocado oil
- 1 medium yellow onion, peeled and diced
- 2 garlic cloves, minced
- 1 medium sweet potato, cut into cubes (peeling not necessary)

- 1/2 pound lean ground turkey
- 1/2 teaspoon salt
- 1 teaspoon Italian seasoning blend

Directions:

1. Attach the oil and allow it to heat for 1 minute. Add the onion and cook until softened, about 5 minutes. Attach the garlic and cook for an additional 30 seconds.
2. Add the sweet potato, turkey, salt, and Italian seasoning and cook for another 5 minutes.

Nutrition:
Calories: 172
Fat: 9 g
Protein: 12 g
Sodium: 348 mg
Fiber: 1 g
Carbs: 10 g
Sugar: 3 g

212. Chicken Tenders with Honey Mustard Sauce

Preparation Time: 5 minutes
Cooking Time: 10 minutes
Servings: 4
Ingredients:

- 1 pound chicken tenders
- 1 tablespoon fresh thyme leaves
- 1/2 teaspoon salt
- 1/4 teaspoon black pepper
- 1 tablespoon avocado oil
- 1 cup chicken stock
- 1/4 cup Dijon mustard
- 1/4 cup raw honey

Directions:

1. Dry the chicken tenders with a towel and then season them with thyme, salt, and pepper.
2. Attach the oil and let it heat for 2 minutes. Add the chicken tenders and seer them until brown on both sides, about 1 minute per side. Press the Cancel button.
3. Remove the chicken tenders and set them aside. Add the stock to the pot. Use a spoon to scrape up any small bits from the bottom of the pot.
4. Set the steam rack in the inner pot and place the chicken tenders directly on the rack.

5. While the chicken is cooking, prepare the sauce.
6. In a bowl, combine the Dijon mustard and honey then stir to combine.
7. Serve the chicken tenders with the honey mustard sauce.

Nutrition:
Calories: 223
Fat: 5 g
Protein: 22 g
Sodium: 778 mg
Fiber: 0 g
Carbs: 19 g
Sugar: 18 g

213. Chicken Breasts with Cabbage and Mushrooms

Preparation Time: 10 minutes
Cooking Time: 18 minutes
Servings: 4
Ingredients:

- 2 tablespoons avocado oil
- 1 pound sliced Baby Bella mushrooms
- 1 ½ teaspoon salt, divided
- 2 garlic cloves, minced
- 8 cups chopped green cabbage
- 1 ½ teaspoon dried thyme
- 1/2 cup chicken stock
- 1 ½ pound boneless, skinless chicken breasts

Directions:

1. Add the oil. Allow it to heat for 1 minute. Attach the mushrooms and 1/4 teaspoon of salt. Saute until they have cooked down and released their liquid, about 10 minutes.
2. Add the garlic and saute for another 30 seconds. Press the Cancel button.
3. Attach the cabbage, 1/4 teaspoon of salt, thyme, and the stock to the inner pot. Stir to combine.
4. Dry the chicken breasts and sprinkle both sides with the remaining salt. Place on top of the cabbage mixture.
5. Transfer to plates and spoon the juices on top.

Nutrition:
Calories: 337
Fat: 10 g
Protein: 44 g

Sodium: 1,023 mg
Fiber: 4 g
Carbs: 14 g
Sugar: 2 g

214. Duck with Bok Choy

Preparation Time: 15 minutes
Cooking Time: 12 minutes
Servings: 6
Ingredients:

- 2 tablespoons coconut oil
- 1 onion, sliced thinly
- 2 teaspoons fresh ginger, grated finely
- 2 minced garlic cloves
- 1 tablespoon fresh orange zest, grated finely
- 1/4 cup chicken broth
- 2/3 cup fresh orange juice
- 1 roasted duck, meat picked
- 3 pounds bok choy leaves
- 1 orange, peeled, seeded and segmented

Directions:

1. In a sizable skillet, melt the coconut oil on medium heat. Attach the onion, saute for around 3 minutes. Add ginger and garlic then saute for about 1-2 minutes.
2. Stir in the orange zest, broth and orange juice.
3. Add the duck meat and cook for around 3 minutes.
4. Transfer the meat pieces to a plate. Add the bok choy and cook for about 3-4 minutes.
5. Divide the bok choy mixture into serving plates and top with duck meat.
6. Serve with the garnishing of orange segments.

Nutrition:
Calories: 290
Fat: 4 g
Fiber: 6 g
Carbs: 8 g
Protein: 14 g

215. Beef with Mushroom and Broccoli

Preparation Time: 60 minutes
Cooking Time: 12 minutes
Servings: 4

Ingredients:
For Beef Marinade:

- 1 garlic clove, minced
- 1 piece fresh ginger, minced
- Salt and freshly ground black pepper
- 3 tablespoons white wine vinegar
- 3/4 cup beef broth
- 1 pound flank steak, trimmed and sliced into thin strips

For Vegetables:

- 2 tablespoons coconut oil
- 2 garlic cloves
- 3 cups broccoli rabe
- 4 ounces shiitake mushrooms
- 8 ounces cremini mushrooms

Directions:

1. For the marinade:
2. In a substantial bowl, mix all ingredients except the beef. Add it and coat with the marinade generously. Refrigerate to soak for around 1/4 hour.
3. In a substantial skillet, warm oil on medium-high heat.
4. Detach the beef from the bowl, reserving the marinade.
5. For the Vegetables:
6. Attach the beef and garlic and cook for about 3-4 minutes or till browned.
7. In the same skillet, add the reserved marinade, broccoli and mushrooms. Cook for approximately 3-4 minutes.
8. Set in the beef and cook for about 3-4 minutes.

Nutrition:
Calories: 200
Carbs: 31 g
Cholesterol: 93 mg
Fat: 4 g
Protein: 10 g
Fiber: 2 g

216. Beef with Zucchini Noodles

Preparation Time: 15 minutes
Cooking Time: 9 minutes
Servings: 4
Ingredients:

- 1 teaspoon fresh ginger, grated
- 2 medium garlic cloves, minced

- 1/4 cup coconut aminos
- 2 tablespoons fresh lime juice
- 1 ½ pound NY strip steak, trimmed and sliced thinly
- 2 medium zucchini, spiralized with blade C
- Salt to taste
- 3 tablespoons essential olive oil
- 2 medium scallions, sliced
- 1 teaspoon red pepper flakes, crushed
- 2 tablespoons fresh cilantro, chopped

Directions:
1. In a big bowl, merge ginger, garlic, coconut aminos and lime juice. Add the beef and coat with the marinade generously. Refrigerate to soak for approximately 10 minutes.
2. Set zucchini noodles over a large paper towel and sprinkle with salt.
3. Keep aside for around 10 minutes.
4. In a big skillet, heat oil on medium-high heat. Attach the scallions and red pepper flakes then saute for about 1 minute.
5. Attach the beef with the marinade and stir fry for around 3-4 minutes or till browned.
6. Stir in the fresh cilantro, then add the zucchini and cook for approximately 3-4 minutes.
7. Serve hot.

Nutrition:
Calories: 1366
Carbs: 166 g
Cholesterol: 6 mg
Fat: 67 g
Protein: 59 g
Fiber. 41 g

217. Spiced Ground Beef

Preparation Time: 10 minutes
Cooking Time: 22 minutes
Servings: 5
Ingredients:
- 2 tablespoons coconut oil
- 2 whole cloves
- 2 whole cardamoms
- 1 (2 inches) piece cinnamon stick
- 2 bay leaves
- 1 teaspoon cumin seeds
- 2 onions, chopped
- Salt to taste

- 1/2 tablespoon garlic paste
- 1/2 tablespoon fresh ginger paste
- 1 pound lean ground beef
- 1 ½ teaspoon fennel seeds powder
- 1 teaspoon ground cumin
- 1 ½ teaspoon red chili powder
- 1/8 teaspoon ground turmeric
- Freshly ground black pepper, to taste
- 1 cup coconut milk
- 1/4 cup water
- 1/4 cup fresh cilantro, chopped

Directions:
1. In a sizable pan, warm oil on medium heat. Mix cloves, cardamoms, cinnamon stick, bay leaves and cumin seeds; cook for about 20 seconds.
2. Attach the onion and 2 pinches of salt then saute for about 3-4 minutes.
3. Add the garlic-ginger paste and stir fry for about 2 minutes.
4. Attach the beef and cook for about 4-5 minutes, entering pieces using the spoon. Stir in spices and cook.
5. Set in the coconut milk and water; cook for about 7-8 minutes. Flavor with salt and take away from the heat.
6. Serve hot using the garnishing of cilantro.

Nutrition:
Calories: 216
Protein: 8.83 g
Fat: 11.48 g
Carbs: 21.86 g

218. Ground Beef with Veggies

Preparation Time: 60 minutes
Cooking Time: 22 minutes
Servings: 4
Ingredients:
- 1-2 tablespoons coconut oil
- 1 red onion,
- 2 red jalapeño peppers
- 2 minced garlic cloves
- 1 pound lean ground beef
- 1 small head broccoli, chopped
- 1/2 head cauliflower
- 3 carrots, peeled and sliced
- 3 celery ribs

- Chopped fresh thyme, to taste
- Dried sage, to taste
- Ground turmeric, to taste
- Salt and freshly ground black pepper

Directions:
1. In a large skillet, dissolve the coconut oil on medium heat.
2. Stir in the onion, jalapeño peppers and garlic. Saute for about 5 minutes.
3. Attach the beef and cook for around 4-5 minutes, entering pieces using the spoon.
4. Add the remaining ingredients and cook, stirring occasionally for about 8-10 minutes.
5. Serve hot.

Nutrition:
Calories: 141
Cholesterol: 50 mg
Carbs: 6 g
Fat: 1 g
Sugar: 3 g
Fiber: 2 g

219. Ground Beef with Greens and Tomatoes

Preparation Time: 15 minutes
Cooking Time: 15 minutes
Servings: 4
Ingredients:

- 1 tablespoon organic olive oil
- 1/2 white onion, chopped
- 2 garlic cloves, finely chopped
- 1 jalapeño pepper, finely chopped
- 1 pound lean ground beef
- 1 teaspoon ground coriander
- 1 teaspoon ground cumin
- 1/2 teaspoon ground turmeric
- 1/2 teaspoon ground ginger
- 1/2 teaspoon ground cinnamon
- 1/2 teaspoon ground fennel seeds
- Salt and freshly ground black pepper
- 8 fresh cherry tomatoes, quartered
- 8 collard green leaves, stemmed and chopped
- 1 teaspoon fresh lemon juice

Directions:
1. In a big skillet, warm oil on medium heat.
2. Add the onion and saute for approximately 4 minutes.
3. Stir in the garlic and jalapeño pepper. Saute for approximately 1 minute.
4. Attach the beef and spices; cook for approximately 6 minutes breaking into pieces while using a spoon.
5. Set in tomatoes and greens. Cook, stirring gently for about 4 minutes.
6. Whisk in lemon juice and take away from the heat.

Nutrition:
Calories: 444
Fat: 15 g
Carbs: 20 g
Fiber: 2 g
Protein: 37 g

Chapter 14. Dinner low fiber

220. Italian Styled Stuffed Zucchini Boats

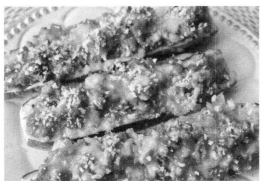

Preparation Time: 10 minutes
Cooking Time: 25 minutes
Servings: 2
Ingredients:

- 6 large zucchini
- 1/2 tablespoon olive oil
- Kosher salt
- Freshly ground black pepper
- 1/4 teaspoon garlic powder
- 1 small yellow onion, diced
- 2 garlic cloves, minced
- 1 pound ground turkey
- 1 (28 ounces) can crush tomatoes
- 4 ounces Mozzarella cheese, shredded
- 1 ounce Parmesan cheese, freshly grated
- Flat-leaf parsley for garnishing
- Cooking spray

Directions:

1. Turn your oven on and allow to preheat up to 425°F and lightly grease a 9x13-inch baking dish with cooking spray.
2. Divide the zucchini in half lengthwise and then scoop out the seeds. Brush with olive oil and season with salt, pepper and garlic powder.
3. Roast in the prepared dish for 20 minutes, or until it begins to soften.
4. Meanwhile, saute the onions and garlic in 1/2 tablespoon of olive oil over medium-high heat in a large skillet.
5. Cook for 3-4 minutes, then add the ground turkey and brown. Attach the tomatoes and bring them to a boil.
6. Reduce the heat to medium and then let simmer until the zucchini are done. Stir in 1/2 teaspoon salt and pepper to taste.
7. Set to bake for about 5 minutes or at least until the Mozzarella cheese you added has melted, about 3-5 minutes.
8. Serve hot, garnished with Parmesan cheese and parsley.

Nutrition:
Calories: 2981
Fat: 7 g
Carbs: 14 g
Fiber: 2 g
Protein: 25 g

221. Chicken Cutlets

Preparation Time: 10 minutes
Cooking Time: 15 minutes
Servings: 4
Ingredients:

- 4 teaspoons red wine vinegar
- 2 teaspoons minced garlic cloves
- 2 teaspoons dried sage leaves
- 1 pound chicken breast cutlets
- Salt and pepper, to taste
- 1/4 cup refined white flour
- 2 teaspoons olive oil

Directions:

1. Set a good amount of plastic wrap on the kitchen counter; sprinkle with half the combined sage, garlic and vinegar.
2. Put the chicken breast on the plastic wrap; sprinkle with the rest of the vinegar mixture. Season lightly with pepper and salt.
3. Secure the chicken with the second sheet of plastic wrap. Use a kitchen mallet to pound the breast until it is flattened. Let stand 5 minutes.
4. Set the chicken on both sides with flour. In a skillet, heat the oil over medium heat.
5. Add half of the chicken breast and cook for 1 ½ minute or until it is browned on the bottom.
6. Turn on the other side and let it cook for 3 minutes.
7. Remove the chicken breast and place it on an oven-proof serving plate so that you can keep warm.

8. Reduce the liquid by half. Pour the mixture over the chicken breast; serve immediately.

Nutrition:
Calories: 549
Fat: 6 g
Carbs: 7 g
Fiber: 1 g
Protein: 114 g

222. Slow Cooker Salsa Turkey

Preparation Time: 8 minutes
Cooking Time: 7 hours
Servings: 4
Ingredients:
- 2 pounds turkey breasts, boneless and skinless
- 1 cup salsa
- 1 cup small tomatoes, diced, canned choose low-sodium
- 2 tablespoons taco seasoning
- 1/2 cup celery, finely diced
- 1/2 cup carrots, shredded
- 3 tablespoons low-fat sour cream

Directions:
1. Add the turkey to your slow cooker. Season it with taco seasoning then top with salsa and vegetables.
2. Add in 1/2 cup of water. Set to cook on low for 7 hours (internal temperature should be 165°F when done).
3. Shred the turkey with 2 forks, add in sour cream and stir. Enjoy.

Nutrition:
Calories: 178
Fat: 4 g
Carbs: 7 g
Fiber: 2 g
Protein: 27 g

223. Sriracha Lime Chicken and Apple Salad

Preparation Time: 10 minutes
Cooking Time: 15 minutes
Servings: 4
Ingredients:
- Sriracha Lime Chicken:
- 2 organic chicken breasts
- 3 tablespoons sriracha
- 1 lime, juiced
- 1/4 teaspoon fine sea salt
- 1/4 teaspoon freshly ground pepper
- Fruit Salad:
- 4 apples, peeled, cored and diced
- 1 cup organic grape tomatoes
- 1/3 cup red onion, finely chopped
- Lime Vinaigrette:
- 1/3 cup light olive oil
- 1/4 cup apple cider vinegar
- 2 limes, juiced
- A dash of fine sea salt

Directions:
1. Use salt and pepper to season the chicken on both sides. Spread on the sriracha and lime and let sit for 20 minutes.
2. Cook the chicken per side over medium heat, or until done. Grill the apple with the chicken.
3. Meanwhile, whisk together the dressing and season to taste.
4. Arrange the salad, topping it with red onion and tomatoes.
5. Serve as a side to the chicken and apple.

Nutrition:
Calories: 484
Fat: 28 g
Carbs: 32 g
Fiber: 8 g
Protein: 30 g

224. Pan-Seared Scallops with Lemon-Ginger Vinaigrette

Preparation Time: 10 minutes
Cooking Time: 10 minutes
Servings: 2
Ingredients:
- 1 pound sea scallops
- 1 tablespoon extra-virgin olive oil
- 1/4 teaspoon sea salt
- 2 tablespoons lemon-ginger vinaigrette
- A pinch of freshly ground black pepper

Directions:
1. Heat the olive oil in a non-stick skillet or pan over medium-high heat until it starts shimmering.

2. Add the scallops to the skillet or pan after seasoning them with pepper and salt. Cook for 3 minutes per side or until the fish is only opaque.
3. Serve with a dollop of vinaigrette on top.

Nutrition:
Calories: 280
Fat: 16
Carbs: 5 g
Sugar: 1 g
Fiber: 0 g
Protein: 29 g
Sodium: 508 mg

225. Roasted Salmon and Asparagus

Preparation Time: 5 minutes
Cooking Time: 15 minutes
Servings: 2
Ingredients:

- 1 tablespoon extra-virgin olive oil
- 1 pound salmon, cut into two fillets
- 1/2 lemon zest and slices
- 1/2 pound asparagus spears, trimmed
- 1 teaspoon sea salt, divided
- 1/8 teaspoon freshly cracked black pepper

Directions:

1. Preheat the oven to 425°F.
2. Stir the asparagus with half of salt and olive oil. At the base of a roasting tray, spread in a continuous sheet.
3. Season the salmon with salt and pepper. Place the asparagus on top of the skin-side down.
4. Lemon zest should be sprinkled over the asparagus, salmon, and lemon slices. Set them over the top.
5. Roast for around 15 minutes until the flesh of the fish is opaque, in the preheated oven.

Nutrition:
Calories: 308
Fat: 18 g
Carbs: 5 g
Sugar: 2 g
Fiber: 2 g
Protein: 36 g
Sodium: 542 mg

226. Orange and Maple-Glazed Salmon

Preparation Time: 15 minutes
Cooking Time: 15 minutes
Servings: 2
Ingredients:

- 1 orange zest
- 1 tablespoon low-sodium soy sauce
- 2 (4-6 ounces) salmon fillets, pin bones removed
- 1 orange juice
- 2 tablespoons pure maple syrup
- 1 teaspoon garlic powder

Directions:

1. Preheat the oven to 400°F.
2. Set the orange juice and zest, soy sauce, maple syrup, and garlic powder in a little shallow bowl.
3. Place the salmon parts in the dish flesh-side down. Allow resting 10 minutes for marinating.
4. Put the salmon on a rimmed baking dish, skin-side up, and bake for 15 minutes, or until the flesh is opaque.

Nutrition:
Calories: 297
Fat: 11
Carbs: 18 g
Sugar: 15 g
Fiber: 1 g
Protein: 34 g
Sodium: 528 mg

227. Cod with Ginger and Black Beans

Preparation Time: 10 minutes
Cooking Time: 15 minutes
Servings: 2
Ingredients:

- 2 (6 ounces) cod fillets
- 1/2 teaspoon sea salt, divided
- 3 minced garlic cloves
- 2 tablespoons chopped fresh cilantro leaves
- 1 tablespoon extra-virgin olive oil
- 1/2 tablespoon grated fresh ginger
- 2 tablespoons freshly ground black pepper
- 1/2 (14 ounces) can black beans, drained

Directions:

1. Heat the olive oil in a big non-stick skillet or pan over medium-high heat until it starts shimmering.
2. Half of the salt, ginger, and pepper are used to season the fish. Cook for around 4 minutes per side in the hot oil until the fish is opaque. Detach the cod from the pan and place it on a plate with aluminum foil tented over it.
3. Add the garlic to the skillet or pan and return it to the heat. Cook for 30 seconds while continuously stirring.
4. Mix the black beans and the remaining salt. Cook, stirring regularly, for 5 minutes.
5. Add the cilantro and serve the black beans on top of the cod.

Nutrition:
Calories: 419
Fat: 2 g
Carbs: 33 g
Sugar: 1 g
Fiber: 8 g
Protein: 50 g
Sodium: 605 mg

228. Halibut Curry

Preparation Time: 10 minutes
Cooking Time: 10 minutes
Servings: 2
Ingredients:

- 1 teaspoon ground turmeric
- 1 pound halibut, skin, and bones removed, cut into 1-inch pieces
- 1/2 (14 ounces) can coconut milk
- 1/8 teaspoon ground black pepper
- 1 tablespoon extra-virgin olive oil
- 1 teaspoon curry powder
- 2 cups no-salt-added chicken broth
- 1/4 teaspoon sea salt

Directions:

1. Heat the olive oil in a non-stick skillet or pan over medium-high heat until it starts shimmering.
2. Add the curry powder and turmeric to a bowl. To bloom the spices, cook for 2 minutes, stirring continuously.
3. Stir in the halibut, coconut milk, chicken broth, pepper, and salt. Lower the heat to medium-low and bring to a simmer. Cook,

stirring regularly, for 6-7 minutes, or until the fish is opaque.

Nutrition:
Calories: 429
Fat: 47 g
Carbs: 5 g
Sugar: 1 g
Fiber: 1 g
Protein: 27 g
Sodium: 507 mg

229. Chicken Cacciatore

Preparation Time: 10 minutes
Cooking Time: 20 minutes
Servings: 2
Ingredients:

- 1 pound skinless chicken, cut into bite-size pieces
- 1/4 cup black olives, chopped
- 1/2 teaspoon onion powder
- A pinch of freshly ground black pepper
- 1 tablespoon extra-virgin olive oil
- 1 (28 ounces) can crushed tomatoes, drained
- 1/2 teaspoon garlic powder
- 1/4 teaspoon sea salt

Directions:

1. Heat the olive oil in a non-stick skillet or pan over medium-high heat until it starts shimmering.
2. Cook until the chicken is browned.
3. Add the tomatoes, garlic powder, olives, salt, onion powder, and pepper, then stir to combine. Cook, stirring regularly, for 10 minutes.

Nutrition:
Calories: 305
Fat: 11 g
Carbs: 34 g
Sugar: 23 g
Fiber: 13 g
Protein: 19 g
Sodium: 1.171 mg

230. Chicken and Bell Pepper Saute

Preparation Time: 5 minutes
Cooking Time: 15 minutes

Servings: 2

Ingredients:

- 1 chopped bell pepper
- 1 pound skinless chicken breasts, cut into bite-size pieces
- 1 ½ tablespoon extra-virgin olive oil
- 1/2 chopped onion
- 3 minced garlic cloves
- 1/8 teaspoon ground black pepper
- 1/4 teaspoon sea salt

Directions:

1. Heat the olive oil in a non-stick skillet or pan over medium-high heat until it starts shimmering.
2. Add the onion, red bell pepper, and chicken. Cook, stirring regularly, for 10 minutes.
3. Stir in the salt, garlic, and pepper in a mixing bowl. Cook for 30 seconds while continuously stirring.

Nutrition:

Calories: 179
Fat: 13 g
Carbs: 6 g
Sugar: 3 g
Fiber: 1 g
Protein: 10 g
Sodium: 265 mg

231. Chicken Salad Sandwiches

Preparation Time: 15 minutes
Cooking Time: 0 minutes
Servings: 2
Ingredients:

- 2 tablespoons anti-inflammatory mayonnaise
- 1 tablespoon chopped fresh tarragon leaves
- 1 cup chicken, chopped, cooked and skinless (from 1 rotisserie chicken)
- 1/2 minced red bell pepper
- 1 teaspoon Dijon mustard
- 4 slices whole-wheat bread
- 1/4 teaspoon sea salt

Directions:

Combine the chicken, red bell pepper, mayonnaise, mustard, tarragon, and salt in a medium mixing bowl.

Spread on 2 pieces of bread and top it with the remaining bread.

Nutrition:

Calories: 315
Fat: 9 g
Carbs: 30 g
Sugar: 6 g
Fiber: 4 g
Protein: 28 g
Sodium: 677 mg

232. Rosemary Chicken

Preparation Time: 15 minutes
Cooking Time: 20 minutes
Servings: 2
Ingredients:

- 1 tablespoon extra-virgin olive oil
- 1 pound chicken breast tenders
- 1 tablespoon chopped fresh rosemary leaves
- 1/8 teaspoon ground black pepper
- 1/4 teaspoon sea salt

Directions:

1. Preheat the oven to 425°F.
2. Set the chicken tenders on a baking sheet with a rim. Sprinkle with salt, rosemary, and pepper after brushing them with olive oil.
3. For 15-20 minutes, keep in the oven, just before the juices run clear.

Nutrition:

Calories: 389
Fat: 20 g
Carbs: 1 g
Sugar: 0 g
Fiber: 1 g
Protein: 49 g
Sodium: 381 mg

233. Gingered Turkey Meatballs

Preparation Time: 10 minutes
Cooking Time: 10 minutes
Servings: 2
Ingredients:

- 1/2 cup shredded cabbage
- 1/2 tablespoon grated fresh ginger
- 1/2 teaspoon onion powder
- 1 pound ground turkey
- 2 tablespoons chopped fresh cilantro leaves
- 1/2 teaspoon garlic powder

- 1/4 teaspoon sea salt
- 1 tablespoon olive oil
- A pinch of freshly ground black pepper

Directions:
1. Combine the cabbage, turkey, cilantro, ginger, onion powder, garlic powder, pepper, and salt in a big mixing bowl. Mix well. Make 10 (3/4 inch) meatballs out of the turkey mixture.
2. Heat the oil in a big non-stick skillet or pan over medium-high heat until it starts shimmering.
3. Cook for about 10 minutes, rotating the meatballs while they brown and you are done.

Nutrition:
Calories: 408
Fat: 26 g
Carbs: 4 g
Sugar: 1 g
Fiber: 1 g
Protein: 47 g
Sodium: 426 mg

234. Turkey and Kale Saute
Preparation Time: 15 minutes
Cooking Time: 35 minutes
Servings: 2
Ingredients:
- 1 pound ground turkey breast
- 1/2 chopped onion
- 1/2 teaspoon sea salt
- 3 minced garlic cloves
- 1 tablespoon extra-virgin olive oil
- 1 cup stemmed and chopped kale
- 1 tablespoon fresh thyme leaves
- A pinch of freshly ground black pepper

Directions:
1. Heat the olive oil in a big non-stick skillet or pan over medium-high heat until it starts shimmering.
2. Add the turkey, onion, kale, thyme, pepper, and salt. Cook, crumbling the turkey with a spoon until it browns, for about 5 minutes.
3. Garlic can be included now. Cook for 30 minutes while continuously stirring.

Nutrition:
Calories: 413

Fat: 20 g
Carbs: 7 g
Sugar: 1 g
Fiber: 1 g
Protein: 50 g
Sodium: 358 mg

235. Turkey with Bell Peppers and Rosemary
Preparation Time: 15 minutes
Cooking Time: 10 minutes
Servings: 2
Ingredients:
- 1 chopped red bell peppers
- 1 pound boneless, skinless turkey breasts, cut into bite-size pieces
- 1/4 teaspoon sea salt
- 2 minced garlic cloves
- 2 tablespoons extra-virgin olive oil
- 1/2 chopped onion
- 1 tablespoon chopped fresh rosemary leaves
- A pinch of freshly ground black pepper

Directions:
1. Heat the olive oil in a non-stick skillet or pan over medium-high heat until it starts shimmering.
2. Add the onion, red bell peppers, rosemary turkey, salt, and pepper. Cook until the turkey is cooked and the veggies are soft.
3. Garlic can be included now. Cook for an additional 30 seconds.

Nutrition:
Calories: 303
Fat: 14 g
Carbs: 15 g
Sugar: 10 g
Fiber: 2 g
Protein: 30 g
Sodium: 387 mg

236. Mustard and Rosemary Pork Tenderloin
Preparation Time: 15 minutes
Cooking Time: 15 minutes
Servings: 2
Ingredients:
- 2 tablespoons Dijon mustard
- 2 tablespoons fresh rosemary leaves

- 1/4 teaspoon sea salt
- 1/2 (1 ½ pound) pork tenderloin
- 1/4 cup fresh parsley leaves
- 3 garlic cloves
- 1 ½ tablespoon extra-virgin olive oil
- 1/8 teaspoon ground black pepper

Directions:
1. Preheat the oven to 400°F.
2. Combine the mustard, parsley, garlic, olive oil, rosemary, pepper, and salt in a blender or food processor. Pulse 20 times in 1-second intervals before a paste emerges. Rub the tenderloin with the paste and place it on a rimmed baking sheet.
3. Bake the pork for around 15 minutes or until an instant-read meat thermometer, reads 165°F.
4. Allow resting for 5 minutes before slicing and serving.

Nutrition:
Calories: 362
Fat: 18 g
Carbs: 5 g
Sugar: 1 g
Fiber: 2 g
Protein: 2 g
Sodium: 515 mg

237. Thin-Cut Pork Chops with Mustardy Kale

Preparation Time: 10 minutes
Cooking Time: 25 minutes
Servings: 2
Ingredients:
- 1 teaspoon sea salt, divided
- 2 tablespoons Dijon mustard, divided
- 1/2 finely chopped red onion
- 1 tablespoon apple cider vinegar
- 2 thin-cut pork chops
- 1/8 teaspoon ground black pepper, divided
- 1 ½ tablespoon extra-virgin olive oil
- 2 cups stemmed and chopped kale

Directions:
1. Preheat the oven to 425°F.
2. Half of salt and pepper are used to season the pork chops. Place them on a rimmed baking sheet and spread 1 tablespoon of mustard over them. Bake for 15 minutes

until an instant-read meat thermometer detects a temperature of 165°F.
3. When the pork cooks, heat the olive oil in a big non-stick skillet or pan over medium-high heat until it starts shimmering.
4. Add the red onion and kale. Cook, stirring regularly, for around 7 minutes, or until the veggies soften.
5. Whisk together the remaining tablespoon of mustard, the remaining half salt, the cider vinegar, and the remaining pepper in a wide mixing bowl. Toss with the kale. Cook for 2 minutes, stirring occasionally.

Nutrition:
Calories: 504
Fat: 39 g
Carbs: 10 g
Sugar: 1 g
Fiber: 2 g
Protein: 28 g
Sodium: 755 mg

238. Beef Tenderloin with Savory Blueberry Sauce

Preparation Time: 10 minutes
Cooking Time: 15 minutes
Servings: 2
Ingredients:
- 1 teaspoon sea salt, divided
- 2 tablespoons extra-virgin olive oil
- 1/4 cup tawny port
- 1 ½ tablespoon very cold butter, cut into pieces
- 2 beef tenderloin fillets, about 3⁄4 inch thick
- 1/8 teaspoon ground black pepper, divided
- 1 finely minced shallot
- 1 cup fresh blueberries

Directions:
1. Half salt and pepper are to be used to season the beef.
2. Heat the olive oil in a big skillet or pan over medium-high heat until it starts shimmering.
3. Add the seasoned steaks to the pan. Cook per side until an instant-read meat thermometer detects an internal temperature of 130°F. Set aside on a plate of aluminum foil tented over it.

4. Get the skillet or pan back up to heat. Add the port, shallot, blueberries, and the remaining salt and pepper to the pan. Scrape some browned pieces off the bottom of the skillet or pan with a wooden spoon. Set the heat to medium-low and bring to a simmer. Cook, stirring from time to time, and gently crushing the blueberries for around 4 minutes or until the liquid has reduced by half.

5. Set in the butter 1 slice at a time. Toss the meat back into the skillet or pan. Mix it once with the sauce to coat it. The rest of the sauce can be spooned over the meat before serving.

Nutrition:
Calories: 554
Fat: 32 g
Carbs: 14 g
Sugar: 8 g
Fiber: 2 g
Protein: 50 g
Sodium: 632 mg

239. Ground Beef Chili with Tomatoes

Preparation Time: 10 minutes
Cooking Time: 15 minutes
Servings: 2
Ingredients:

- 1/2 chopped onion
- 1 (14 ounces) can kidney beans, drained
- 1/2 pound extra-lean ground beef
- 1 (28 ounces) can chopped tomatoes, undrained
- 1/2 tablespoon chili powder
- 1/4 teaspoon sea salt
- 1/2 teaspoon garlic powder

Directions:

1. Cook the beef and onion in a big pot over medium-high heat for around 5 minutes.
2. Add the kidney beans, tomatoes, garlic powder, chili powder, salt, and stir to combine. Bring to boil, then reduce to low heat.
3. Cook for 10 minutes, stirring occasionally.

Nutrition:
Calories: 890

Fat: 20 g
Carbs: 63 g
Sugar: 13 g
Fiber: 17 g
Protein: 116 g
Sodium: 562 mg

240. Fish Taco Salad with Strawberry Avocado Salsa

Preparation Time: 20 minutes
Cooking Time: 15 minutes
Servings: 2
Ingredients:
For the salsa:

- 2 hulled and diced strawberries
- 1/2 diced small shallot
- 2 tablespoons finely chopped fresh cilantro
- 2 tablespoons freshly squeezed lime juice
- 1/8 teaspoon cayenne pepper
- 1/2 diced avocado
- 2 tablespoons canned black beans, rinsed and drained
- 1 thinly sliced green onions
- 1/2 teaspoon finely chopped peeled ginger
- 1/4 teaspoon sea salt

For the fish salad:

- 1 teaspoon agave nectar
- 2 cups arugula
- 1 tablespoon extra-virgin olive or avocado oil
- 1/2 tablespoon freshly squeezed lime juice
- 1 pound light fish (halibut, cod, or red snapper), cut into 2 fillets
- 1/4 teaspoon ground black pepper
- 1/2 teaspoon sea salt

Directions:
For the salsa:
Preheat the grill, whether it's gas or charcoal.

1. Add the avocado, beans, strawberries, shallot, cilantro, green onions, salt, ginger, lime juice, and cayenne pepper in a medium mixing cup. Put aside after mixing until all the components are well combined.

For the fish salad:

2. Whisk the agave, oil, and lime juice in a small bowl. Set the arugula with the vinaigrette in a big mixing bowl.

3. Season the fish fillets with pepper and salt. Grill the fish for 7-9 minutes over direct high heat, flipping once during cooking. The fish should be translucent and quickly flake.
4. Place 1 cup of arugula salad on each plate to eat. Cover each salad with a fillet and a heaping spoonful of salsa.

Nutrition:
Calories: 878
Fat: 26 g
Carbs: 53 g
Sugar: 15 g
Fiber: 18 g
Protein: 119 g
Sodium: 582 mg

241. Beef and Bell Pepper Stir-Fry

Preparation Time: 5 minutes
Cooking Time: 10 minutes
Servings: 2
Ingredients:

- 3 scallions, white and green parts, chopped
- 1 tablespoon grated fresh ginger
- 2 minced garlic cloves
- 1/2 pound extra-lean ground beef
- 1 chopped red bell peppers
- 1/4 teaspoon sea salt

Directions:
1. Cook the beef for around 5 minutes in a big non-stick skillet or pan until it browns.
2. Add the scallions, ginger, red bell peppers, and salt. Cook, stirring occasionally, for around 4 minutes or until the bell peppers are tender.
3. Garlic can be included now. Cook for 30 seconds while continuously stirring. Switch off the flame, and you are done.

Nutrition:
Calories: 599
Fat: 19 g
Carbs: 9 g
Sugar: 4 g
Fiber: 2 g
Protein: 97 g
Sodium: 520 mg

242. Veggie Pizza with Cauliflower-Yam Crust

Preparation Time: 5 minutes
Cooking Time: 1hour 10 minutes
Servings: 2
Ingredients:

- 1/2 medium peeled and chopped garnet yam
- 1 teaspoon sea salt, divided
- 1/2 tablespoon coconut oil, plus more for greasing pizza stone
- 1/4 cup sliced cremini mushrooms
- 1/4 medium head cauliflower, cut into small florets
- 1/2 tablespoon dried Italian herbs
- 1/2 cup flour brown rice
- 1/2 sliced small red onion
- 1/2 zucchini or yellow summer squash
- 2 tablespoons vegan pesto
- 1/2 cup spinach

Directions:
1. Heat the oven to 400°F or preheat the pizza stone in case you have one.
2. Set a big pot with 1 inch of water, place a steamer basket. Put the yam and cauliflower in the steamer basket and steam for 15 minutes, or until both are quickly pricked with a fork. If you overcook the vegetables, they can get too soggy.
3. Place the vegetables in a food blender or processor and pulse until smooth. Blend in the Italian herbs and half a teaspoon of salt until smooth. Set the mixture in a big mixing bowl. Gradually whisk in the flour until it is well mixed.
4. Use coconut oil to grease the pizza stone or a pizza plate. In the middle of the pizza stone, pile the cauliflower mixture. Spread the pizza dough uniformly in a round or circular way (much like frosting) with a spatula until the crust is around 1/8 inches thick.
5. Bake for around 45 minutes. To get the top crispy, switch on the broiler and cook it for 2 minutes.
6. In a medium skillet or pan, melt the coconut oil over medium heat. Cook for 2 minutes after adding the onion. Add the squash, mushrooms, and the remaining ingredients to a large mixing bowl. Saute for 3-4 minutes

with a quarter teaspoon of salt. Detach the spinach from the heat as soon as it starts to wilt.

7. Evenly, plate the pesto around the pizza crust. Over the pesto, spread the sautéed vegetables. It's time to slice the pizza and eat it.

Nutrition:
Calories: 329
Fat: 17 g
Carbs: 9 g
Sugar: 3 g
Fiber: 5 g
Protein: 37 g
Sodium: 430 mg

243. Toasted Pecan Quinoa Burgers

Preparation Time: 5 minutes
Cooking Time: 30 minutes
Servings: 2
Ingredients:
- 2 cups vegetable broth, divided
- 1 teaspoon sea salt
- 2 tablespoons sesame seeds
- 1/2 teaspoon dried oregano
- 1/4 cup canned black beans,
- 2 tablespoons pecans
- 1/2 cup quinoa, rinsed and drained
- 1/4 cup sunflower seeds
- 1/2 teaspoon ground cumin
- 1/2 shredded carrot
- Freshly ground black pepper
- 1/2 thinly sliced avocado
- 1/2 teaspoon coconut or sunflower oil

Directions:
1. Preheat the oven to 375°F.
2. Roast the pecans for 5-7 minutes on a baking sheet.
3. In a big saucepan, bring 1 cup of broth, quinoa, and salt to a boil over medium-high heat. Set the heat to a minimum, cover, and cook for 20 minutes, stirring occasionally.
4. In a food processor, grind the pecans, cumin, sesame seeds, sunflower seeds, and oregano to a medium-coarse texture.
5. Combine a half cup of quinoa, carrots, nut mixture, and beans in a big mixing bowl.

Slowly, pour the remaining cup of broth, constantly stirring, before the paste becomes tacky. Season with pepper and salt as per taste.

6. Set the mixture into 2 (1/2-inch thick) patties and cook, refrigerate them right away.
7. In a big skillet or pan over medium-high heat, melt the coconut oil. Cook for around 2 minutes on either side. Carry on for the remaining patties in the same manner. Avocado slices can be placed on top of the burgers.

Nutrition:
Calories: 432
Fat: 12 g
Carbs: 12 g
Sugar: 5 g
Fiber: 3 g
Protein: 57 g
Sodium: 566 mg

244. Sizzling Salmon and Quinoa

Preparation Time: 10 minutes
Cooking Time: 30 minutes
Servings: 2
Ingredients:
- 1/2 teaspoon extra-virgin olive oil
- 1/2 cup quinoa, rinsed and drained
- 1/4 pound sliced chanterelle mushrooms
- 1/2 cup frozen small peas
- 1 tablespoon chopped fresh basil
- 1 head garlic
- 1 ½ cup mushroom broth, divided
- 1 tablespoon coconut oil
- 1/2 cup shredded brussels sprouts
- 1 tablespoon nutritional yeast
- 1/2 tablespoon dried oregano
- Sea salt and freshly ground black pepper
- 1/4 pound salmon, skin, and bones removed, cut into 1-inch cubes

Directions:
1. Preheat the oven to 350°F.
2. Detach the top of the garlic head to reveal the cloves. Cover the head in foil and drizzle with olive oil. Set in the oven for 50 minutes to roast.

3. Meanwhile, in a big saucepan, mix 1 cup of broth and the quinoa. Set to a boil over high heat, then reduce to low heat, cover, and simmer without stirring for 20 minutes. To make this dish, measure 1/4 cup of quinoa, reserving any leftovers for another use.

4. Heat the coconut oil in a big skillet or pan over medium heat. Saute for 5 minutes, or before the mushrooms release liquid and become tender.

5. Cook for 3 minutes with the brussels sprouts, adding up to 1/4 cup of broth if required to keep the mushrooms and sprouts from sticking to the skillet or pan.

6. Saute for 5 minutes, stirring regularly, with the peas, basil, nutritional yeast, and oregano.

7. Toss the salmon in the pan to mix. Squeeze the garlic cloves gently into it. Cook, secured, for 4-5 minutes, stirring periodically.

8. Stir in the remaining 1/4 cup of broth and 1/4 cup of quinoa in the skillet or pan until all is well mixed. Season with pepper and salt to taste.

9. Serve.

Nutrition:
Calories: 599
Fat: 20 g
Carbs: 10 g
Sugar: 4 g
Fiber: 6 g
Protein: 88 g
Sodium: 662 mg

Chapter 15. Dinner high fiber

245. Grilled Pear Cheddar Pockets

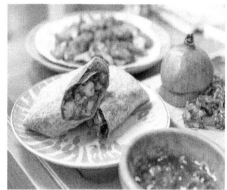

Preparation time: 15 minutes
Serving: 1
Ingredients:

- Dijon mustard – 2 tsp
- Whole grain flatbread – half
- Cheddar cheese – 2 slices
- Arugula – ¼ cup
- Red pear – 1/3, cored and cut into thick slices

Directions:

1. Spread mustard over the inner side of the flatbread pocket.
2. Place cheese slices and fold them. Then, add pear slices and arugula.
3. Place it into the skillet and cook for 3 to 4 minutes.

Nutrition:
Calories; 223kcal, fat ; 8.6g, Carbohydrate; 28.6g, Protein; 11.3g, Fiber; 6.8g

246. Chicken and Apple Kale Wraps

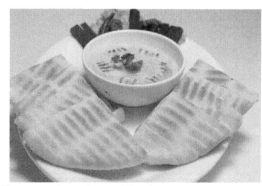

Preparation time: 10 minutes
Serving: 1
Ingredients:

- Mayonnaise – 1 tbsp
- Dijon mustard – 1 tsp
- Kale leaves – three
- Chicken breast – three ounces, thinly sliced, cooked
- Red onion – six slices, thin
- Apple – one, cut into nine slices

Directions:
Combine the mustard and mayonnaise into the bowl. Spread onto the kale leaves—top with one-ounce chicken, three slices of apples, and two slices of onion. Then, roll each kale leaf. Cut in half.
Nutrition:
Calories; 370kcal, fat ; 13.7g, Carbohydrate; 34.1g, Protein; 29.3g, Fiber; 6g

247. Cauliflower Rice Pilaf

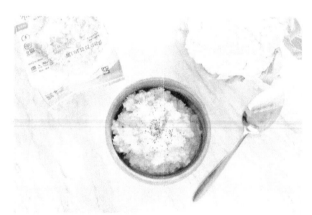

Preparation time: 10 minutes
Cooking time: 10 minutes
Serving: 1
Ingredients:

- Cauliflower florets – six cups
- Extra-virgin olive oil – three tbsp
- Garlic – two cloves, minced
- Salt – half tsp
- Almonds – ¼ cup, toasted, sliced
- Herbs – ¼ cup, chopped
- Lemon zest – 2 tsp

Directions:

1. Add cauliflower florets into the food processor and blend until chopped.
2. Add oil into the skillet and place it over medium-high flame.
3. Then, add garlic and cook for a half-minute.

4. Add cauliflower rice and season with salt. Let cook for three to five minutes.
5. Remove from the flame.
6. Add lemon zest, herbs, and almonds and stir well.

Nutrition:
Calories; 114kcal, fat ; 9.2g, Carbohydrate; 6.7g, Protein; 3g, Fiber; 2.8g

248. Fresh Herb and Lemon Bulgur Pilaf

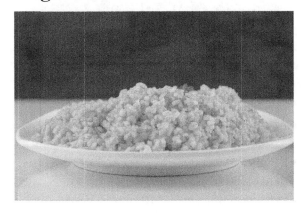

Preparation time: 10 minutes
Cooking time: 40 minutes
Serving: 6
Ingredients:
- Extra-virgin olive oil – 2 tbsp
- Onion – two cups, chopped
- Garlic – one clove, chopped
- Bulgur – 1 ½ cups
- Ground turmeric – half tsp
- Ground cumin – half tsp
- Vegetable or chicken broth – 2 cups, low-sodium
- Carrot – 1 ½ cups, chopped
- Fresh ginger – 2 tsp, grated or chopped
- Salt – one tsp
- Fresh dill – ¼ cup, chopped
- Fresh mint – ¼ cup, chopped
- Parsley – ¼ cup, chopped
- Lemon juice – three tbsp
- Walnuts – half cup, chopped, toasted

Directions:
1. Add oil into the skillet and place it over medium flame.
2. Add onion and cook for 12 to 18 minutes.
3. Add garlic and cook for one minute.

4. Then, add cumin, turmeric, and bulgur and cook for one minute.
5. Add salt, ginger, carrot, and broth and bring to a boil over medium0high flame, about 15 minutes.
6. Remove from the flame.
7. Let rest for five minutes.
8. Add lemon juice, parsley, dill, and mint into the pilaf and stir well.
9. Garnish with walnuts.

Nutrition:
Calories; 273kcal, fat ; 11.7g, Carbohydrate; 38.8g, Protein; 7.3g, Fiber; 7.7g

249. Corn Chowder

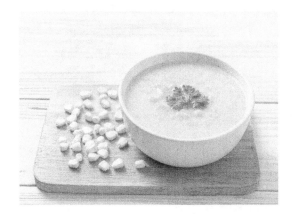

Preparation time: 10 minutes
Cooking time: 5 hours
Serving: 6
Ingredients:
- Yellow split peas – ¾ cup, split
- Chicken broth – 28 ounces, low-sodium
- Water – one cup
- Corn kernels – 12 ounces, frozen
- Red sweet peppers – half cup, chopped and roasted
- Green chilies – 4 ounces, diced
- Ground cumin – one tsp
- Dried oregano – half tsp, crushed
- Dried thyme – half tsp, crushed
- Cream cheese – ½ cup

Directions:
1. Rinse split peas underwater.
2. Mix the thyme, oregano, cumin, chilies, red peppers, corn, water, split peas, and chicken broth and cook on high heat for five to six hours.
3. Let cool it for ten minutes.

4. Transfer two cups of soup into the food processor and blend until smooth.

Add pureed soup into the slow cooker. Then, add cream cheese and whisk to combine—Cook for five minutes.

Serve!

Nutrition:

Calories; 222kcal, fat ; 7.5g, Carbohydrate; 29.8g, Protein; 10.5g, Fiber; 7.7g

250. Strawberry and Rhubarb Soup

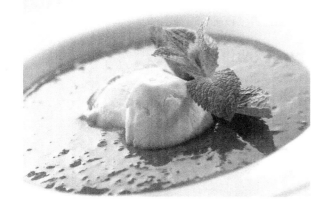

Preparation time: 5 minutes
Cooking time: 30 minutes
Serving: 4
Ingredients:

- Rhubarb – four cups
- Water – three cups
- Strawberries – 1 ½ cups, sliced
- Sugar – ¼ cup
- Salt – 1/8 tsp
- Mint or basil – 1/3 cup, chopped
- Ground pepper – to taste

Directions:

1. Add three cups of water and rhubarb into the saucepan.
2. Cook for five minutes until softened.
3. Transfer it to the bowl.
4. Add 2-inch ice water into the bowl and keep it aside with rhubarb.
5. Place it into the fridge for twenty minutes.
6. Transfer the rhubarb to the blender. Then, add salt, sugar, and strawberries and blend until smooth.
7. Place it back in the bowl. Add basil or mint.

Serve!

Nutrition:

Calories; 95kcal, fat ; 0.5g, Carbohydrate; 23.1g, Protein; 1.6g, Fiber; 3.5g

251. Chicken Sandwiches

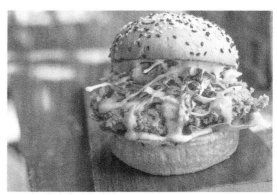

Preparation time: 5 minutes
Cooking time: 30 minutes
Serving: 4
Ingredients:

- Red onion – four slices
- Red sweet pepper – one, seeded and quartered
- Chicken breast – six ounces, boneless, cut in half, horizontally
- Multi-grain sandwich round – four, split
- Basil pesto – 2 tbsp
- Kalamata olives – 2 tbsp, pitted and chopped
- Mozzarella cheese – 1/3 cup, shredded
- Feta cheese – ¼ cup, low-fat, crumbled

Directions:

1. Heat the skillet over medium flame.
2. Let coat with pepper and red onion with non-stick cooking spray.
3. Add it to the pan and cook for six to eight minutes.
4. Remove from the skillet. Let coat the chicken with non-stick cooking spray.
5. Add chicken to the grill pan and cook for three to five minutes.
6. Remove from the skillet.
7. Pull chicken into shreds. Cut pepper into strips.
8. To assemble the sandwiches: Spread the pesto onto the sandwich and sprinkle with olives. Place grilled onion slices. Top with pepper strips.
9. Place chicken over it. Sprinkle with feta cheese and mozzarella cheese.
10. Then, place skillet over medium-low flame.
11. Place the sandwich into the skillet and cook for three to four minutes.

12. Flip and cook for three to four minutes.
13. Serve!

Nutrition:
Calories; 296kcal, fat ; 10g, Carbohydrate; 27.7g, Protein; 25.8g, Fiber; 6.2g

252. Tex-Mex Bean Tostadas

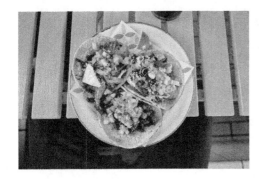

Preparation time: 10 minutes
Cooking time: 15 minutes
Serving: 4
Ingredients:

- Tostada shells – four
- Pinto beans – 16 ounces, rinsed and drained
- Salsa – half cup, prepared
- Chipotle seasoning – ½ tsp
- Cheddar cheese – ½ cup, shredded
- Iceberg lettuce – 1 ½ cups
- Tomato – one cup, chopped
- Lime wedges – one

Instruction:

1. Preheat the oven to 350 degrees Fahrenheit.
2. Place tostada shells onto the baking sheet and bake for three to five minutes.
3. Meanwhile, mix the seasoning, salsa, and bean into the bowl.
4. Mash the mixture with a potato masher.
5. Then, divide the bean mixture between tostada shells.
6. Top with half of the cheese. Bake for five minutes.
7. Top with chopped tomato and shredded lettuce.
8. Then, place the remaining cheese and lime wedges.

Nutrition:
Calories; 230kcal, fat ; 6g, Carbohydrate; 33g, Protein; 12g, Fiber; 6g

253. Fish Tacos

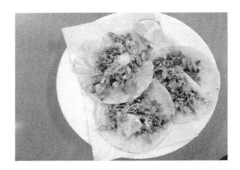

Preparation time: 10 minutes
Cooking time: 15 minutes
Serving: 4
Ingredients:

- Tilapia fillets – 1lb
- Extra-virgin olive oil – 2 tsp
- Chipotle seasoning blend – 2 tsp
- Coleslaw mix – 2 cups
- Salad dressing – 2 tbsp, ranch
- Whole wheat tortillas – eight
- Avocado – half, thinly sliced
- Cilantro leaves – ¼ cup
- Lime – one, quartered

Directions:

1. Preheat the oven to 450 degrees Fahrenheit.
2. Place fillets onto the baking dish and brush the fish with oil.
3. Sprinkle with seasoning.
4. Bake for four to six minutes.
5. Meanwhile, mix the dressing and coleslaw into a bowl. Keep it aside.
6. Flake the fish into big chunks and place them into the tortillas.
7. Top with lime, cilantro, avocado, and coleslaw mixture.

Nutrition:
Calories; 341kcal, fat ; 12g, Carbohydrate; 30.5g, Protein; 29.5g, Fiber; 21.2g

254. Cucumber Almond Gazpacho

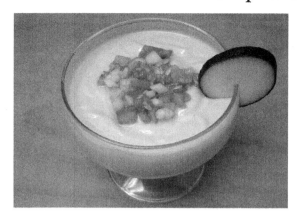

Preparation time: 20 minutes
Chill time: 2 hours
Serving: 5
Ingredients:

- English cucumbers – two
- Yellow bell pepper – two cups, chopped
- Whole wheat bread – 2 cups
- Unsweetened almond milk – 1 ½ cups
- Almonds – ½ cup, toasted, slivered
- Olive oil – five tsp
- White-wine vinegar – 2 tsp
- Garlic – one clove
- Salt – half tsp

Directions:

1. Dice unpeeled cucumber and mix with half a cup bell pepper.
2. Peel the remaining cucumbers and cut them into chunks.
3. Add remaining bell pepper, peeled cucumber, salt, garlic, vinegar, oil, six tbsp of almonds, almond milk, and bread into the blender and blend until smooth. Let chill for two hours.
4. Garnish with the remaining 2 tbsp almonds.
5. Drizzle with oil.

Nutrition:
Calories; 201kcal, fat ; 11.8g, Carbohydrate; 19g, Protein; 6.3g, Fiber; 4.3g

255. Pea and Spinach Carbonara

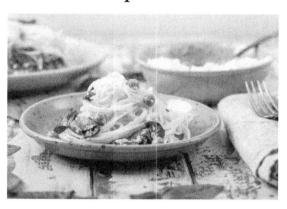

Preparation time: 5 minutes
Cooking time: 15 minutes
Serving: 4
Ingredients:

- Extra-virgin olive oil – 1 ½ tbsp
- Panko breadcrumbs (whole-wheat) – half cup
- Garlic – one clove, minced
- Parmesan cheese – eight tbsp, grated
- Fresh parsley – three tbsp, chopped
- Egg yolks – three
- Egg – one
- Ground pepper – half tsp
- Salt – ¼ tsp
- Tagliatelle or linguine – 9 ounce
- Baby spinach – eight cups
- Peas – one cup

Directions:

1. Add ten cups of water into the pot and boil it over high flame.
2. During this, add oil into the skillet and cook over medium-high flame.
3. Add garlic and breadcrumbs and cook for two minutes until toasted.
4. Transfer it to the small bowl. Add parsley and two tbsp parmesan cheese and keep it aside.
5. Whisk the salt, pepper, egg, egg yolks, and six tbsp parmesan cheese into the bowl.
6. Add pasta to the boiling water and cook for one minute.
7. Add spinach and peas and cook for one minute more until tender.
8. Save ¼ cup of the cooking water for your next use. Drain it and place it into the bowl.

9. Whisk the reserved cooking water into the egg mixture, add to the pasta, and toss to combine.
10. Top with breadcrumb mixture and serve!

Nutrition:
Calories; 430kcal, carbohydrates; 54.1g, protein; 20.2g, fat; 14.5g, fiber; 8.2g

256. Sautéed Broccoli with Peanut Sauce

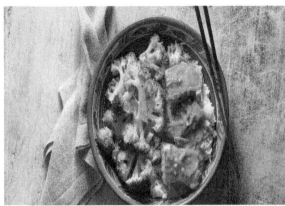

Preparation time: 5 minutes
Cooking time: 10 minutes
Serving: 6
Ingredients:

- Broccoli florets – eight cups
- Sesame oil – two tbsp, toasted
- Red bell pepper – one cup, sliced
- Yellow onion – half cup, sliced
- Garlic – three cloves, chopped
- Peanut butter – three tbsp
- Tamari – 2 ½ tbsp, low-sodium
- Rice vinegar – two tbsp
- Brown sugar –one tbsp
- Cornstarch – one tsp
- Sesame seeds – one tbsp, toasted

Directions:

1. Add water into the pot and boil it. Then, add broccoli and cook for three to four minutes until tender.
2. During this, add oil into the skillet and cook over medium-high flame.
3. Add garlic, onion, and bell pepper and cook for three minutes.
4. Add steamed broccoli and cook for three minutes. Stir well.

5. Whisk the cornstarch, sugar, vinegar, tamari, and peanut butter into the bowl. Add vegetables and stir well.
6. Let cook for one minute. Top with sesame seeds.
7. Serve and enjoy!

Nutrition:
Calories; 154kcal, carbohydrates; 12g, protein; 6g, fat; 9.7g, fiber; 3.4g

257. Edamame lettuce wraps burgers

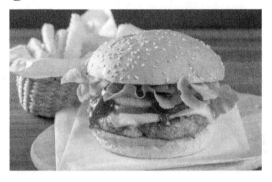

Preparation time: 5 minutes
Cooking time: 25 minutes
Serving: 4
Ingredients:

- Carrots – one cup, julienned
- Lime juice – three tbsp
- Chili-garlic sauce – two tsp
- Shelled edamame – 1 ½ cups, thawed
- Cooked brown rice – one cup
- Peanut butter powder – half cup
- Scallions – ¼ cup, chopped
- Red Thai curry paste – one tbsp
- Peanut oil – three tbsp
- Tamari – two tbsp, low-sodium
- Bibb lettuce – four leaves
- Red onion – one cup, thinly sliced

Directions:

1. Firstly, toss carrots with one tsp chili garlic sauce and two tbsp lime juice and keep it aside.
2. Add tamari, one tbsp oil, curry paste, scallions, edamame rice, and ¼ cup peanut butter powder into the blender and blend until smooth.
3. Shape the mixture into four burgers.

4. Add two tbsp oil into the skillet and cook over medium flame.
5. Add burgers and cook for three to four minutes per side.
6. When done, transfer it to the plate.
7. During this, whisk the one tsp chili garlic sauce, tamari, one tbsp lime juice, and ¼ cup peanut butter powder into the bowl until smooth.
8. Then, drain the carrots. Add marinade to the peanut sauce. Stir well.
9. Wrap burger in lettuce leaves and top with sauce, onions, and carrots.

Nutrition:
Calories; 310kcal, carbohydrates; 31.6g, protein; 14.6g, fat; 14.5g, fiber; 7.6g

258. Pizza stuffed Spaghetti Squash

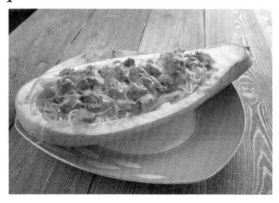

Preparation time: 10 minutes
Cooking time: 1 hour
Serving: 4
Ingredients:
- Spaghetti squash – three pounds, halved lengthwise and seeded
- Water – ¼ cup
- Extra-virgin olive oil – two tbsp
- Onion – one cup, chopped
- Garlic – two cloves, minced
- Mushrooms – eight ounce, sliced
- Bell pepper – one cup, chopped
- No-salt-added crushed tomatoes – two cups
- Italian seasoning – one tsp
- Ground pepper – half tsp
- Crushed red pepper – ¼ tsp, crushed
- Salt – ¼ tsp
- Pepperoni – two ounce, halved

- Part-skim mozzarella cheese – one cup, shredded
- Parmesan cheese – two tbsp, grated

Directions:
1. Preheat the oven to 450 degrees Fahrenheit.
2. Add squash into the microwave-safe dish and then add water.
3. Let microwave it for ten to twelve minutes until tender.
4. Then, place it into the oven and bake for forty to fifty minutes at 400 degrees Fahrenheit.
5. During this, add oil into the skillet and cook over medium flame.
6. Add garlic and onion and cook for three to four minutes.
7. Add bell pepper and mushrooms and cook for five minutes more until tender.
8. Add salt, crushed red pepper, pepper, Italian seasoning, and tomatoes and cook for two minutes.
9. When done, remove from the flame.
10. Add ten to twelve pepperoni halves and cover them with a lid.
11. Scrape the squash from the shells and place it into the bowl.
12. Add salt, pepper, mozzarella, and parmesan cheese and stir well.
13. Add tomato mixture to the bowl and stir well.
14. Place squash shells onto the rimmed baking sheet and divide the filling among the halves, and top with pepperoni and mozzarella cheese. Place it into the oven and bake for fifteen minutes.
15. Let broil it for one to two minutes.
16. Serve and enjoy!

Nutrition:
Calories; 373kcal, carbohydrates; 32.2g, protein; 16.4g, fat; 20.6g, fiber; 7.5g

259. Spinach and Artichoke Dip Pasta

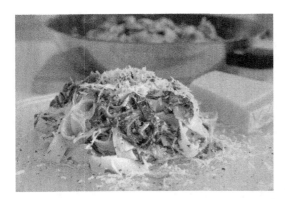

Preparation time: 5 minutes
Cooking time: 15 minutes
Serving: 4
Ingredients:

- Whole-wheat rotini – eight ounce
- Baby spinach – five ounce, chopped
- Cream cheese – four ounce, low-fat, cut into chunks
- Milk – ¾ cup, low-fat
- Parmesan cheese – half cup, grated
- Garlic powder – two tsp
- Ground pepper – ¼ tsp
- Artichoke hearts – 14 ounce, rinsed, squeezed dry and chopped

Directions:
1. Add water into the saucepan and boil it. Add pasta and cook it. Then, drain it.
2. Mix the one tbsp water and spinach into the saucepan and cook over medium flame. Cook for two minutes until wilted.
3. Transfer it to the bowl. Add milk and cream to the pan and whisk it well.
4. Add pepper, garlic powder, and parmesan cheese and cook until thickened. Drain spinach and add to the sauce with pasta and artichoke. Cook it well.
5. Then, serve and enjoy!

Nutrition:
Calories; 371kcal, carbohydrates; 56.1g, protein; 16.6g, fat; 9.1g, fiber; 7.9g

260. Grilled Eggplant

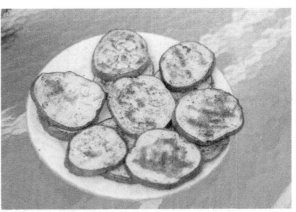

Preparation time: 5 minutes
Cooking time: 40 minutes
Serving: 4
Ingredients:

- Water – four cups
- Cornmeal – one cup
- Butter – one tbsp
- Salt – half tsp
- Plum tomatoes – 1lb, chopped
- Extra-virgin olive oil – four tbsp
- Fresh oregano – two tsp, chopped
- Garlic – one clove, grated
- Ground pepper – half tsp
- Crushed red pepper – ¼ tsp
- Eggplant – 1 ½ lbs, cut into half-inch-thick slices
- Feta cheese – ¼ cup, crumbled
- Fresh basil – half cup, chopped

Directions:
1. Add water into the saucepan and boil it over high flame.
2. Add cornmeal and whisk it well. Then, lower the heat and cook for thirty-five minutes until tender.
3. When done, remove from the flame. Add salt and butter and stir well.
4. During this, preheat the grill over medium-high heat.
5. Add salt, crushed red pepper, pepper, garlic, oregano, three tbsp oil, and tomatoes into the bowl and toss to combine.
6. Rub eggplant with one tbsp oil and place onto the grill, and cook for four minutes per side. Let cool it for ten minutes.
7. Let chop it and add to the tomatoes.

8. Sprinkle with fresh basil leaves.
9. Place vegetable mixture over the polenta and top with cheese.

Nutrition:
Calories; 354kcal, carbohydrates; 39g, protein; 6.8g, fat; 20.6g, fiber; 8.4g

261. Stuffed potatoes with salsa and beans

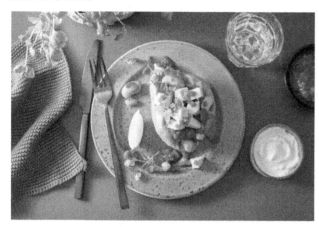

Preparation time: 5 minutes
Cooking time: 20 minutes
Serving: 4
Ingredients:

- Russet potatoes – four
- Fresh salsa – half cup
- Avocado – one, sliced
- Pinto beans – 15 ounce, rinsed, warmed and mashed
- Jalapeños – four tsp, chopped, pickled

Directions:
1. Firstly, pierce potatoes using a fork.
2. Let microwave for twenty minutes over medium heat.
3. Place onto the cutting board and let cool it.
4. Cut to open the potato lengthwise and pinch the ends to expose the flesh and top with jalapeno, beans, avocado, and salsa.
5. Serve and enjoy!

Nutrition:
Calories; 324kcal, carbohydrates; 56.7g, protein; 9.2g, fat; 8g, fiber; 11g

262. Mushroom quinoa veggie Burgers

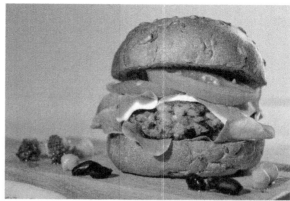

Preparation time: 5 minutes
Cooking time: 25 minutes
Chill time: 1 hour
Serving: 4
Ingredients:

- Portobello mushroom – one, gills removed, chopped
- Black beans – one cup, rinsed, unsalted
- Almond butter – two tbsp, creamy and unsalted
- Canola mayonnaise – three tbsp
- Ground pepper – one tsp
- Smoked paprika – ¾ tsp
- Garlic powder – ¾ tsp
- Salt – half tsp
- Cooked quinoa – half cup
- Old-fashioned rolled oats – ¼ cup
- Ketchup – one tbsp
- Dijon mustard – one tsp
- Extra-virgin olive oil – one tbsp
- Whole-wheat hamburger buns – four, toasted
- Green-leaf lettuce – two leaves, halved
- Tomato – four sliced
- Red onion – four, thinly sliced

Directions:
1. Add salt, half tsp garlic powder, paprika, pepper, one tbsp mayonnaise, almond butter, black beans, and mushrooms into the food processor. Blend until smooth.
2. Transfer it to the bowl. Add oats and quinoa and stir well.
3. Place it into the refrigerator for one hour.
4. During this, whisk the ¼ tsp garlic powder, two tbsp mayonnaise, mustard, and ketchup into the bowl until smooth.
5. Make the mixture into four patties.

6. Add oil into the non-stick skillet and cook over medium-high flame.
7. Fry patties for four to five minutes.
8. Flip and cook for two to four minutes until golden brown.
9. Top burger with onion, tomato, lettuce, and sauce.

Nutrition:
Calories; 395kcal, carbohydrates; 45.9g, protein; 11.6g, fat; 19.8g, fiber; 9.4g

263. Turkey Meatballs

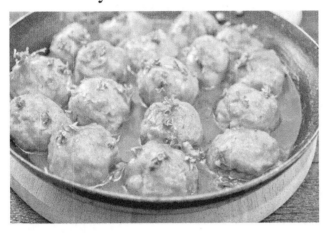

Preparation time: 15 minutes
Cooking time: 25 minutes
Serving: 4
Ingredients:
- Olive oil – one tsp
- Button mushrooms – three cups, sliced
- Egg – one, beaten
- Quick-cooking rolled oats – 1/3 cup
- Parmesan cheese – 1/3 cup, grated
- Garlic – three cloves, minced
- Dried Italian seasoning – two tsp, crushed
- Salt – half tsp
- Ground pepper – ¼ tsp
- Lean ground turkey – 1 ¼ lbs

Directions:
1. Preheat the oven to 400 degrees Fahrenheit.
2. Line a baking pan with foil and coat it with cooking spray.
3. Add oil into the skillet and cook over medium flame.
4. Add mushroom and cook for eight to ten minutes.

5. Transfer it to the blender and blend until chopped.
6. Mix the pepper, salt, Italian seasoning, garlic, parmesan cheese, oats, and egg into the bowl. Add chopped mushrooms and turkey and combine well.
7. Place meat mixture onto the cutting board and cut into thirty squared.
8. Roll each square into the ball, place it onto the pan, and bake for twelve to fifteen minutes.
9. Serve and enjoy!

Nutrition:
Calories; 467kcal, carbohydrates; 49.2g, protein; 36.3g, fat; 16.1g, fiber; 7.6g

264. Sweet Potato Soup

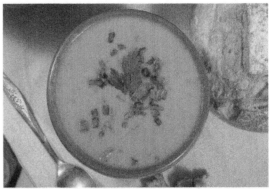

Preparation time: 15 minutes
Cooking time: 30 minutes
Serving: 6
Ingredients:
- Canola oil – ¼ cup
- Corn tortillas – four, halved and thinly sliced
- Salt – ¾ tsp
- Poblano pepper – one, seeded and chopped
- Onion – one, chopped
- Chili powder – two tbsp
- Chicken broth or vegetable broth – four cups
- Sweet potatoes – 1 ½ lbs, peeled and cut into half-inch pieces
- Tomatoes – 14 ounce, unsalted, pitted, diced
- Black beans – 15 ounce, low-sodium, rinsed
- Lime juice – three tbsp
- Radishes – three, halved and thinly sliced
- Pumpkin seeds – ¼ cup, roasted, unsalted
- Queso fresco – half cup, crumbled

- Avocado – one, chopped

Directions:

Add oil into the pot and cook over medium flame.

1. Add tortilla strips and cook for five minutes until crispy.
2. Transfer it to the plate lined with a paper towel using a slotted spoon.
3. Sprinkle with ¼ tsp salt.
4. Add half tsp salt, chili powder, onion, and poblano, and cook for two minutes until softened.
5. Add tomatoes, beans, broth, and sweet potatoes and simmer for twenty minutes.
6. Add lime juice into the soup and top with tortilla strips, avocado, queso fresco, pepitas, and radish slices. Stir well.
7. Serve and enjoy!

Nutrition:

Calories; 412kcal, carbohydrates; 45g, protein; 13.5g, fat; 21.6g, fiber; 11.7g

265. Minestrone Soup

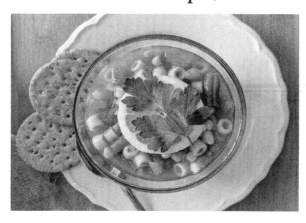

Preparation time: 5 minutes
Cooking time: 25 minutes
Serving: 6
Ingredients:

- Garlic – five cloves, minced
- Extra-virgin olive oil – three tbsp
- Whole-grain rustic bread – one cup, cubed
- Leek – one cup, chopped, white and light green parts only
- Carrots – one cup, chopped
- Vegetable broth – three cups
- Water – three cups
- Kosher salt – ¾ tsp
- Ditalini pasta – one cup

- Zucchini – ten ounce, halved lengthwise and thinly sliced
- Cannellini beans – 15 ounce, unsalted, rinsed
- Kale – three cups, chopped
- Frozen peas – one cup, thawed
- Ground pepper – half tsp

Directions:

1. Preheat the oven to 350 degrees Fahrenheit.
2. Add two tbsp oil and garlic and cook over medium flame for three to four minutes.
3. Add bread and toss to combine. Place mixture onto the baking sheet and bake for eight to ten minutes.
4. During this, add one tbsp oil into the pot and cook over medium-high flame. Add carrots and leek and cook for five to six minutes.
5. Add salt, water, and broth and cover with a lid and boil it over high flame. Add pasta and lower the heat to medium-high and cook for five minutes. Add zucchini and cook for five minutes until al dente.
6. Add pepper, peas, kale, and beans and stir well. Let cook for two minutes.
7. Place soup into the six bowls. Top with croutons.

Nutrition:

Calories; 267kcal, carbohydrates; 38.7g, protein; 9.7g, fat; 8.6g, fiber; 7.2g

266. Lentil Soup

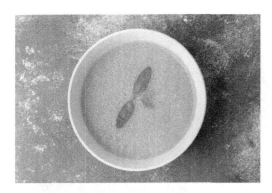

Preparation time: 5 minutes
Cooking time: 1 hour
Serving: 6
Ingredients

- Onion – one, chopped
- Olive oil – ¼ cup
- Carrots – two, diced
- Celery – two stalks, chopped
- Garlic – two cloves, minced
- Dried oregano – one tsp
- Bay leaf – one
- Dried basil – one tsp
- Crushed tomatoes – 14.5 ounces
- Dry lentils – two cups
- Water – eight cups
- Spinach – half cup, rinsed and thinly sliced
- Vinegar – two tbsp
- Salt and ground black pepper – to taste

Directions:
1. Add oil into the pot and cook over medium flame.
2. Add celery, carrots, and onions and cook until tender.
3. Add basil, oregano, bay leaf, garlic, and stir well and cook for two minutes.
4. Add tomatoes, water, and lentils and stir well. Let boil it.
5. Lower the heat and simmer for one hour.
6. Add spinach and cook until wilted.
7. Add pepper, salt, and vinegar and stir well.

Nutrition:
Calories; 349kcal, carbohydrates; 48.2g, protein; 18.3g, fat; 10g, fiber; 22.1g

267. Grilled Corn Salad

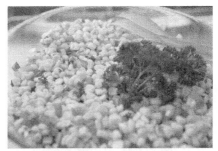

Preparation time: 15 minutes
Cooking time: 10 minutes
Additional time: 45 minutes
Servings: 6
Ingredients:

- Freshly shucked corn – six ears
- Green pepper – one, diced
- Tomatoes – two plum, diced
- Red onion – ¼ cup, diced
- Fresh cilantro – half bunch, chopped
- Olive oil – two tsp
- Salt and ground black pepper – to taste

Directions:
1. Preheat the grill over medium heat. Oil the grate.
2. Place corn onto the grill and cook for ten minutes and keep it aside.
3. Let cool it. Cut the kernels off the cob and place them into the medium bowl.
4. Mix the olive oil, cilantro, onion, diced tomato, green pepper, and corn kernels and sprinkle with pepper and salt.
5. Toss to combine. Let stand for thirty minutes.
6. Serve and enjoy!

Nutrition:
Calories; 103kcal, carbohydrates; 19.7g, protein; 3.4g, fat; 2.8g, fiber; 3.3g

268. Kale Soup

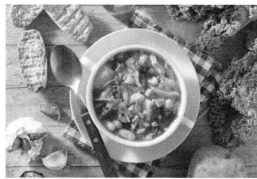

Preparation time: 25 minutes
Cooking time: 30 minutes
Servings: 8
Ingredients:

- Olive oil – two tbsp
- Yellow onion – one, chopped
- Garlic – two, tbsp
- Kale – one bunch, stems removed and leaves chopped
- Water – six cups
- Vegetable bouillon – six cubes
- Tomatoes – 15 ounce, diced
- White potatoes – six, peeled and cubed
- Cannellini beans – 30 ounce, drained
- Italian seasoning – one tbsp
- Dried parsley – two tbsp
- Salt and pepper – to taste

Directions:
Add olive oil into the pot and heat it.
Add garlic and onion and cook until softened.
Add kale and stir, and cook for two minutes.
Add parsley, Italian seasoning, beans, potatoes, tomatoes, vegetable bouillon, and water and stir well. Let simmer for twenty-five minutes.
Sprinkle with pepper and salt.

Nutrition:
Calories; 277kcal, carbohydrates; 50.9g, protein; 9.6g, fat; 4.5g, fiber; 10.3g

269. Pasta Fagioli

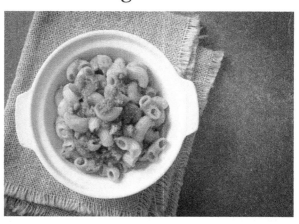

Preparation time: 10 minutes
Cooking time: 30 minutes
Servings: 4
Ingredients:

- Olive oil – one tbsp
- Carrot – one, diced
- Celery – one stalk, diced
- Onion – one, diced, thinly sliced
- Garlic – half tsp, chopped
- Tomato sauce – eight ounce,
- Chicken broth – 14 ounce
- Ground black pepper – to taste
- Dried parsley – one tbsp
- Dried basil leaves – half tbsp
- Cannellini beans – 15 ounce, drained and rinsed
- Ditalini pasta – 1 ½ cups

Directions:
Add olive oil into the saucepan and heat it over medium flame.
Add onion, celery, and carrot and cook until fragrant.
Add garlic and cook it well. Add basil, parsley, pepper, chicken broth, and tomato sauce and simmer for twenty minutes.
Add salt and water into the pot and boil it. Add ditalini pasta and cook for eight minutes until al dente. Let drain it.
Add beans to the sauce mixture and simmer for a few minutes.
When pasta is done, add bean mixture and sauce and stir well.
Serve and enjoy!
Nutrition:

Calories; 338kcal, carbohydrates; 60.7g, protein; 13.4g, fat; 5.1g, fiber; 9.4g

270. Sweet Potato Gnocchi

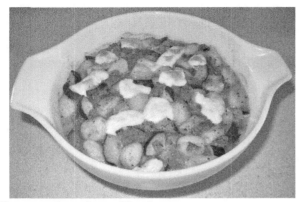

Preparation time: 30 minutes
Cooking time: 35 minutes
Servings: 4
Ingredients:

- Sweet potatoes – eight ounce
- Garlic – one clove, pressed
- Salt – half tsp
- Ground nutmeg – half tsp
- Egg – one
- All-purpose flour – two cups

Directions:

1. Preheat the oven to 350 degrees Fahrenheit.
2. Let bake for thirty minutes until softened.
3. When done, remove it from the oven and keep it aside to cool.
4. When cooled, peel and mash them and add them to the bowl.
5. Add egg, nutmeg, salt, and garlic and mix it well.
6. Add flour and combine it well.
7. Add water and salt into the pot and boil it.
8. To prepare the gnocchi: Roll the dough onto the floured surface and cut it into sections.
9. Add pieces into the boiled water and cook until they floated on the surface.
10. When done, remove and serve!
11. Top with cream sauce or butter.

Nutrition:
Calories; 346kcal, carbohydrates; 71.1g, protein; 9.9g, fat; 2.1g, fiber; 5.2g

271. Bean and Ham Soup

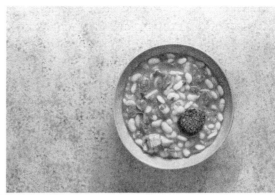

Preparation time: 25 minutes
Cooking time: 10 hours
Servings: 12
Ingredients:

- Sweet potatoes – two
- Garlic – one clove, pressed
- Salt – half tsp
- Ground nutmeg – half tsp
- Egg – one
- All-purpose flour – two cups
- Bean mixture – 20 ounce, soaked overnight
- Ham bone – one
- Ham – 2 ½ cups, cubed
- Onion – one, chopped
- Celery – three stalks, chopped
- Carrots – five, chopped
- Tomatoes – 14.5 ounce, diced, with liquid
- Vegetable juice – 12 fluid ounce, low-sodium
- Vegetable broth – three cups
- Worcestershire sauce – two tbsp
- Dijon mustard – two tbsp
- Chili powder – one tbsp
- Bay leaves – three
- Ground black pepper – one tsp
- Dried parsley – one tbsp
- Lemon juice – three tbsp
- Chicken broth – seven cups, low-sodium
- Kosher salt – one tsp

Directions:

1. Add soaked beans into the pot, and then add water until it covers the beans. Let boil it on low flame for thirty minutes. Then, drain it.
2. Add vegetable broth, vegetable juice, tomatoes, carrots, celery, onion, ham, and ham bone and sprinkle with lemon juice,

parsley, pepper, bay leaf, chili powder, Dijon mustard, and Worcestershire sauce.

3. Add chicken broth and simmer on low flame for eight hours.
4. Add more chicken broth as required. Remove the ham bone and sprinkle with salt.
5. Let simmer for two hours more.
6. Discard bay leaves.

Nutrition:
Calories; 260kcal, carbohydrates; 37.9g, protein; 17.3g, fat; 3.6g, fiber; 14.8g

Chapter 16. Simple recipes

272. Pork Menudo

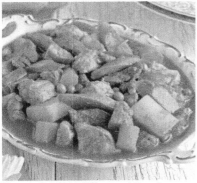

Preparation Time: 10 minutes
Cooking Time: 1 hour
Servings: 6
INGREDIENTS:

- 2 lbs. pork
- 1/4 lb. pig liver
- One cup of potatoes diced
- One-piece carrot cubed
- 1/2 cup of soy sauce
- 1/2 pieces lemon
- One-piece onion chopped
- Three cloves garlic minced
- One teaspoon sugar
- 3/4 cup of tomato sauce
- One cup of water
- Four pieces of hotdogs sliced diagonally
- Two tbsp cooking oil
- 2 to 3 pieces dried bay leaves
- Salt and pepper to taste

DIRECTIONS:
1. In a bowl, mix meat, soy sauce, and lemon. Marinate for a minimum of 1 hour.
2. Heat oil in a casserole
3. Saute onion and garlic.
4. Add pork marinated—Cook for five to seven minutes.
5. Pour in the sauce of the tomato and water and add the bay leaves.
6. Cook and cook for 30 minutes, depending on the harshness of the pork. Note: Add water as required.
7. Add liver and hot dogs to it.
8. Five minutes of cooking time.

9. Put in pomme of cabbage, carrots, sugar, salt, and pepper. Stir and cook for eight to twelve minutes.
NUTRITION: Calories 523 Fat 37g Carbohydrates 12g Protein 33g

273. Pork Caldereta Recipe
Preparation Time: 5 minutes
Cooking Time: 1 hour
Servings: 6
INGREDIENTS:

- 2 lbs. Pork sliced into cubes
- One-piece Knorr Pork cube
- Eight oz. tomato sauce
- ¾ cup of green olives
- One-piece red bell pepper sliced
- One-piece green bell pepper sliced
- Two pieces of potatoes cubed
- Two pieces carrot sliced
- One-piece onion chopped
- Three clove garlic chopped
- 1 1/Two cups of water
- ½ cup of the liver spread
- Three tbsp cooking oil
- Salt and ground black pepper to taste

DIRECTIONS:
1. Heat the oil in a pot.
2. Sprinkle the garlic and onion once the oil gets heated.
3. Add pork. Add pork. Sprinkle till light brown becomes color.
4. Sprinkle with tomato sauce and water. Let boil. Let boil. Cover and cook for 60 minutes in low heat.
5. Add the spread of the liver. Remove and cook for 3 minutes.
6. Put in the carrot and potatoes. Cover and cook for eight to ten minutes.
7. Add olives and peppers to the bell. Five minutes of cooking time.
NUTRITION: Calories 650 Fat 51g Carbohydrates 10g Protein 37g

274. Bicol Express Gising Gising
Preparation Time: 5 minutes
Cooking Time: 30 minutes
Servings: 4
INGREDIENTS:

- 1 lb pork belly sliced

- Two cups of long green beans
- One-piece Knorr Pork cube
- 4 cups of coconut milk
- One-piece onion
- Two thumbs ginger
- Four cloves garlic chopped
- Six pieces chili pepper
- Three 1/Two tbsp shrimp paste
- One tbsp cooking oil
- Ground black pepper to taste

DIRECTIONS:

1. Add the belly of pork. Sear until the fat extracts enough oil.
2. Add onion, garlic, chili pepper, and ginger. Keep cooking until the onion softens.
3. Add the paste of shrimp. Saute 1 minute
4. In the pan, pour coconut milk. Cover and let boil. Let boil.
5. Add pork cube to Knorr. Stir. Cover the pot and adjust the heat to the lowest possible position. Keep cooking until the pork becomes soft.
6. Fill in long green beans—five minutes of cooking time.
7. Season with black pepper ground.

NUTRITION: Calories 1142 Fat 113g Carbohydrates 14g Protein 27g

275. Nilagang Baka Recipe

Preparation Time: 10 minutes
Cooking Time: 1 hour 12 minutes
Servings: 6
INGREDIENTS:

- 2 lbs. beef sirloin cubed
- Two bunches baby bok choy
- One-piece cabbage
- Six pieces Saba banana halved
- Four pieces baking potato quartered
- One-piece white onion halved
- Four stars celery chopped
- One-piece star anise
- 4 cups of beef broth
- 4 cups of water
- Salt and pepper to taste

DIRECTIONS:

1. In a large cooking pot, mix the water and beef broth. Bring to boil. Bring to boil.

2. Fill in the onion, anise star, and celery. Reduce medium heat. Cover the saucepan and keep boiling for 20 minutes.
3. Remove an onion, star anise, and celery using a skimmer or sieve from the boiling liquid. These ingredients can be discarded.
4. Add beef. Add beef. Simmer for 60 to 90 minutes or until tender. If necessary, you can add extra water.
5. Put banana and potatoes in the saba. Cook 10 minutes. Cook 10 min.
6. Cover and disable the heat. Let the saucepan keep covered for 2 to 5 minutes to cook the vegetables.

NUTRITION: Calories 243 Fat 6g Carbohydrates 11g Protein 36g

276. Chicken Afritada Recipe

Preparation Time: 5 minutes
Cooking Time: 45 minutes
Servings: 6
INGREDIENTS:

- 1 ½ lb. Chicken cut into serving pieces
- Two-piece potato cubed
- One-piece carrot sliced
- Eight oz. tomato sauce
- Three pieces hotdog sliced
- ½ cup of green peas
- Three pieces bay leaves
- One-piece red onion chopped
- Two teaspoons garlic minced
- 3 cups of chicken broth
- ½ teaspoon sugar
- Three tbsp cooking oil
- Salt and ground black pepper to taste

DIRECTIONS:

1. Heat the oil in a pot. Sprinkle onion and garlic until the onion is tender.
2. Add chicken. Chicken. Cook 30 seconds. Cook 30 seconds. Turn it over and cook another 30 seconds on the other side.
3. Sprinkle with tomato sauce and chicken broth.
4. Add dried leaves of the bay. Cover the pot for cooking. Continue to cook for 30 minutes on medium heat.
5. Add carrot and hotdogs—three minutes of cooking time.

6. Add potato. Add potato. Cover the saucepan for 8 minutes and cook.
7. Fill in the green peas. Cook 2 minutes. Cook 2 minutes.
NUTRITION: Calories 583 Fat 37 Carbohydrates 25g Protein 37g

277. Chicken Paksiw
Preparation Time: 5 minutes
Cooking Time: 40 minutes
Servings: 6
INGREDIENTS:
- One lb. leftover chicken cut into pieces
- One-piece Knorr Chicken Cube
- One cup of Lechon sauce
- Five clove garlic chopped
- One-piece onion chopped
- One teaspoon whole peppercorn
- Four pieces of dried bay leaves
- 1/2 cup of white vinegar
- 1/4 cup of sugar
- One cup of water
- Salt to taste
- Three tbsp cooking oil

DIRECTIONS:
1. In a pot, heat oil. Onion and garlic saute.
2. When the onion is smooth, add the chicken. Remove and sprinkle for 1 minute.
3. In the pool, add the Lechon sauce and vinegar. Before stirring, let the mixture boil.
4. Place the water in the pan. Let it boil. Let it boil.
5. Add Knorr Chicken Cube, laurel, and whole pepper. Stir. Cover the pot, then adjust the heat to the lowest position. Continue to cook for 35 minutes.
6. Take the pan off the cover. Continue to boil until the sauce evaporates and is halved.
7. Add sugar and sauté with salt.
8. Transfer to a bowl and serve warm rice. Share and take pleasure!
NUTRITION: Calories 441 Fat 29g Carbohydrates 21g Protein 23g

278. Chicken Binagoongan
Preparation Time: 5 minutes
Cooking Time: 45 minutes
Servings: 4-8
INGREDIENTS:

- 2 lbs. chicken cut into serving pieces
- 3 ½ tbsp bagoong
- Five pieces winged bean cigarillos, sliced
- One-piece onion chopped
- Four cloves garlic crushed and chopped
- Two pieces tomato cubed
- Two tbsp white vinegar
- One teaspoon granulated white sugar
- 1 ½ cups of water
- Three tbsp cooking oil
- Three parts Thai chili chopped
- One-piece Serrano pepper sliced
- Ground black pepper to taste

DIRECTIONS:
1. In a pot, heat oil. For 25 seconds, sauce onion.
2. Add garlic. Add garlic. Selle for 30 seconds. For 30 seconds.
3. Add tomato. Tomato. Continue to simmer until tomatoes are tender.
4. In the pan, put the chicken. Saute till the exterior color becomes medium brown.
5. Add bagoong wireless (shrimp paste). Cook 1 minute. Cook 1 minute.
6. Pour into the pan with vinegar. Allow the liquid to boil.
7. Place the water in the pan. Cover and let boil then. Five minutes boil. Boil.
8. Add boobs winged (cigarillos). Cover and then simmer for 30 minutes between low and medium heat.
9. Season with sugar and add paste of shrimp if necessary.
10. Add chili and green pepper for lengthy periods. Three minutes of cooking time.
NUTRITION: Calories 158 Fat 11g Carbohydrates 5g Protein 11g

279. Adobong Kangkong Recipe
Preparation Time: 5 minutes
Cooking Time: 15 minutes
Servings: 4

INGREDIENTS:
- One bunch of Kangkong leaves and stalks separated. Stalks cut into One-inch pieces
- One-piece onion chopped
- One head garlic crushed and chopped

- 1/4 cup of soy sauce
- 1/8 cup of vinegar
- 1/2 cup of water optional
- Three tbsp cooking oil
- Ground black pepper

DIRECTIONS:
1. Heat pan oil. 1.
2. Add garlic. Add garlic. Sprinkle till the color becomes golden brown. Scoop the browned garlic out a quarter and place it in a clean basin. Save this for garnish later.
3. Add onion chopped. Sprinkle till it softens.
4. In the pan, pour the soy sauce and the vinegar. Allow the liquid to boil.
5. Add the stalks of Kangkong. Cook two minutes. Two minutes.
6. Add the leaves of Kangkong. Stir. Keep cooking for 30 to 1 minute. Cover the casserole and heat for 1 minute.
7. Season with black ground pepper. Note: if necessary, you can also add salt.
8. Transfer to a serving bowl, then brown garlic.
9. Serve. Share and take pleasure!

NUTRITION: Calories 169 Fat 14g Carbohydrates 8g Protein 4g

280. Ginisang Labanos Recipe

Preparation Time: 5 minutes
Cooking Time: 30 minutes
Servings: 6
INGREDIENTS:
- One lb. daikon white radish, sliced into thick strips
- One-piece carrot sliced into wide strips
- One-piece tomato cubed
- 3/4 cup of pork thinly sliced
- 3/4 cup of dried shrimp small
- One-piece onion sliced
- Three cloves garlic crushed
- Two teaspoon fish sauce
- 1/2 cup of water
- 1/Two teaspoon ground black pepper
- Two tbsp cooking oil

DIRECTIONS:
1. Heat oil in a casserole
2. Salt onion and garlic
3. Once the onion is tender, throw the tomato into it—three minutes of cooking time.

4. Add pork. Add pork—five minutes of cooking time.
5. Put water in and let it boil—cover and cook for 10 minutes.
6. Add the daikon and carrot to it. Stir. Cover 5 minutes and cook.
7. Add the shrimp, sauce of fish, and black ground pepper. Stir and cook for another 10 minutes.

NUTRITION: Calories 492 Fat 25g Carbohydrates 15g Protein 57g

281. Sizzling Pusit

Preparation Time: 7 minutes
Cooking Time: 20 minutes
Servings: 4
INGREDIENTS:
- Two pieces of squid (giant) cleaned
- One-piece carrot sliced thinly
- One-piece bell pepper cut into squares
- One-piece onion wedged
- ½ teaspoon ginger minced
- ½ cup of celery stalk sliced
- Two tbsp cooking oil
- 1 ½ tbsp margarine
- Salt and ground black pepper to taste
- ½ piece Knorr Shrimp Cube
- One teaspoon Knorr Liquid Seasoning
- 1 ½ teaspoon all-purpose flour
- ¼ cup of banana ketchup
- ¼ cup of cooking wine
- ½ cup of water
- ¼ teaspoon garlic powder
- ½ teaspoon onion powder
- Two tbsp margarine

DIRECTIONS:
1. Melt Two tbsp of margarine in a pot to make the sauce. Add meal. Remove from medium to high heat and continue cooking for 1 minute. Add shrimp cube to Knorr. Continue to whisk until all ingredients are thoroughly mixed. Add the Knorr Liquid Seasoning, banana ketchup, wine, and water to cook. Remove and let boil. Season with powdered garlic and powdered onion. Set aside. Set aside.
2. Heat 2 cooking oil teaspoons in a pan. Sauce ginger and onion until the onion layers are separated.
3. Carrot and celery stir-in. Cook 1 minute. Cook 1 minute.

4.   Add squid and bell pepper. Continue to cook for 2 minutes—season with black pepper and salt.

5.   Heat 1 1/2 margarine tbsp in a metal dish. Add squid and vegetables and pour over the sauce.

NUTRITION: Calories   215   Fat   17g Carbohydrates 12g Protein 2

282. Pork Steak

Preparation Time: 10 minutes
Cooking Time: 50 minutes
Servings: 4
INGREDIENTS:

- 4 pieces pork chops
- Five tbsp soy sauce
- Two pieces of lime
- 1/2 cup of cooking oil
- Two pieces of onions sliced
- 1 1/Two cups of water
- 1/Two teaspoon granulated white sugar

DIRECTIONS:

1.   In a large bowl or resealable bag, mix pork chops, soy sauce, and lime juice. Marinate for a minimum of 1 hour.

2.   Then heat a pan for-in cooking oil.

3.   Pan-fry the medium-heat pork chops for 3 minutes on every side.

4.   Remove oversupply of oil. Pour in and let boil the remaining marinade. Simmer until meat is tender for 45 minutes. Note: Add water as necessary.

5.   Stir in the sugar, salt, and pepper.

6.   Put the onions in and cook for another 3 minutes.

7.   Switch off the heat and transfer to a plate of service.

8.   Serve. Share and take pleasure!

NUTRITION: Calories 265 Fat 28 Carbohydrates 2g Protein 3g

283. Pork Katsu Curry Recipe

Preparation Time: 20 minutes
Cooking Time: 45 minutes
Servings: 4
INGREDIENTS:

- 3 pieces pork chops
- 1 ½ cups of cooking oil
- 3 cups of cooked white rice
- Two cups of water
- Two cups of ice cubes
- 1/4 cup of salt
- Two tbsp brown sugar
- Two pieces of dried bay leaves
- Breading **Ingredients:**
- ½ cup of all-purpose flour
- 1 ½ cup of Panko breadcrumbs
- Two pieces of eggs beaten
- Curry Sauce Ingredients
- One-piece Knorr Pork Cube
- One-piece onion chopped
- One-piece carrot sliced
- One-piece potato cubed
- One teaspoon ginger grated
- One clove garlic grated
- ½ piece apple peeled and grated
- One tbsp curry powder
- One tbsp garam masala
- Five tbsp butter
- Four tbsp all-purpose flour
- Two ¾ cups of water
- Salt and ground black pepper to taste

DIRECTIONS:

1.   Make the salt by putting in a cooking pot all salt ingredients except ice cubes. Let it boil. Let it boil. Mix until sugar and salt are fully diluted. Let it cool down. Let it cool down. Mix the solution of salt and ice cubes.

2.   Arrange pork chops in a resealable plastic bag and then add the ice cubes to the salt solution. Seal the bag. Seal the bag. Do not cool for more than 8 hours.

3.   Melt the curry sauce into a pot with two tbsp of butter. Add onion. Add onion. Cook until the texture is soft. Add ginger and garlic. Remove and add carrot and potato. Keep cooking for 1 minute. Cover for 6 minutes and cook. Set aside. Set aside.

4.   Melt the roux in a cooking pot by melting Three tbsp of butter. Add meal for all purposes. Remove and cook for 4 minutes. Add the curry and garam masala powder. Cook for a minute while stirring. Place 1 3/Two cups of water in the pot. Remove till the mixture thickens. Add pork cube to Knorr. Stir. Add pot contents with onion and potato. Keep cooking for 3 to 5 minutes. Season with black pepper and salt. Set aside. Set aside.

5.   Make pork tonkatsu using running water by rinsing pork. Pat dry with towels of paper.

6.   Heat oil to 350F in a frying saucepan. Dredge a piece of pork chop in the flour while oil is heating. Excess shake-off. Dip in the beaten egg and the breadcrumbs of Panko. Dip again in egg and dredge again in breadcrumbs.

7.   Deep brown pork chop till gold brown is turned out on the outside, and the inside temperature is 145F or above. Remove from the pot and cool. Slice into portions.

8.   Set a cup of rice on a dish. Top with the tonkatsu sliced pork, and then add the curry sauce to the top.

NUTRITION: Calories   5059   Fat   403g Carbohydrates 330g Protein 41g

284. Crispy Kare-Kare

Preparation Time: 15minutes
Cooking Time: 1 hour 30 minutes
Servings: 6
INGREDIENTS:

- 4 lbs. pork belly
- 5 cups of water
- Three tbsp salt
- 3 cups of cooking oil
- 1/2 cup of bagoong alamang
- Kare-Kare Sauce:
- Two cups of roasted peanuts
- One-piece Knorr Pork Cube
- 1/2 cup of annatto seeds
- One-piece onion chopped
- Three cloves garlic minced
- 1 ½ tbsp toasted rice powder
- Two cups of water
- Three tbsp cooking oil
- Vegetable **ingredients:**
- Two bunches pechay
- One-piece eggplant sliced
- 12 pieces string beans
- One cup of banana blossoms sliced

DIRECTIONS:
1.   Prepare pork. Boil water for 35 minutes, continue to boil. Remove the pork from the pot and cook it. Rub salt all over and leave for 5 minutes to stay.

2.   Heat oil in a big pot. When the oil is hot, cook the pork belly (skin side down). Note: Be FOOD! Sprinkle 1 1/Two teaspoon of water on the oil every 3 minutes or until the skin becomes very crisp, golden brown.

3.   Flip the pork and cook until golden brown on the opposite side. Remove pork from the frying saucepan to let the excess oil drain over the wire rack. Set aside. Set aside.

4.   Begin to make the sauce. Grind the peanuts in a food processor until the texture is paste-like. Set aside. Set aside.

5.   Make annatto water for 5 minutes by soaking annatto seeds in boiling water. Stir constantly until the water turns orange deep. Use a kitchen strainer to filter the water. You can then discard the seeds. Set aside. Set aside.

6.   Saute onion and garlic. Add the peanut paste once the onion softens. Remove and cook for 1 minute.

7.   Pour water and mix until the mixture is smooth. Allow the liquid to boil.

8.   Add pork cube Knorr and water annatto. Cover and cook for 3 minutes. Remove the top and heat until the mixture is less than desired. Add toasted powder of rice. Mix thoroughly. Mix well. Turn the heat off. Make sure the saucepan remains warm to the sauce.

9.   Cook the vegetables through the steaming process. Arrange on the steamer string bean, banana flower, and eggplant. Steam 5 minutes. Steam 5 minutes. Add pechay and moisture for 2 to 3 minutes.

10.   Assemble your crispy care by putting in a single plate sauce, steamed veggies, and crispy pork. Serve with alamang rice and bagoong.

NUTRITION: Calories   3096   Fat   305g Carbohydrates 42g Protein 60g

285. Halabos na Hipon with Butter

Preparation Time: 5 minutes
Cooking Time: 10 minutes
Servings: 6
INGREDIENTS:

- One lb. shrimp deveined
- One cup of lemon-lime soda
- Two tbsp butter
- One tbsp parsley chopped
- ½ teaspoon salt

DIRECTIONS:
1.   Then add the shrimp and heat the pan. Stir.

2. Boil, stirring shrimp softly once in a while. Continue to cook until the liquid is halved.

3. Add salt and butter, season with salt. Continue to cook for 1 to 2 minutes.

NUTRITION: Calories 251 Fat 10g Carbohydrates 8g Protein 31g

286. Ginataang Kalabasa at Sitaw

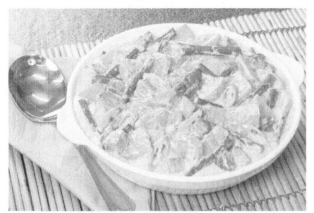

Preparation Time: 5 minutes
Cooking Time: 35 minutes
Servings: 6-8
INGREDIENTS:

- 1 1/2 lbs. squash cubed
- 18 pieces string beans cut into Two-inch pieces
- One-piece Knorr Pork cube
- 3 ounces pork sliced into small pieces, preferably boiled
- 4 cups of coconut milk
- One-piece onion chopped
- Two thumbs ginger sliced into strips
- Five cloves garlic crushed
- ¼ teaspoon ground black pepper
- One tbsp cooking oil
- Fish sauce to taste

DIRECTIONS:

1. Add pork. Pork. Cook till crispy and golden.
2. Sprinkle with garlic, onion, and ginger.
3. Pour the cocoa milk into the pan once the onion softens. Stir. Cover the pot and let the liquid boil. Adjust the heat to medium once you boil and continue to boil for 5 minutes.
4. Add pork cube and squash to Knorr. Continue to cook for 5 minutes.
5. Add beans string—Cook for five to eight minutes.

6. Season with black ground pepper and fish sauce if necessary.

NUTRITION: Calories 512 Fat 38g Carbohydrates 41g Protein 13g

287. Filipino Chicken Macaroni Salad Recipe

Preparation Time: 10minutes
Cooking Time: 35 minutes
Servings: 8
INGREDIENTS:

- One lb. boneless chicken breast
- 1 lb elbow macaroni
- One 1/Two cups of Lady's Choice Mayonnaise
- One can pineapple chunks 20 oz
- 1 1/Two cups of shredded cheddar cheese
- One bottle pimiento 6.5 Ounces chopped
- One cup of carrot chopped
- One-piece green bell pepper chopped
- One cup of raisins
- 1/4 cup of sweet relish
- 1/Two teaspoon garlic powder
- Three teaspoons of salt will be used when boiling chicken and macaroni and as a seasoning
- 1/Four teaspoon ground black pepper
- Water for boiling

DIRECTIONS:

1. Prepare chicken, prepare chicken. Start boiling the chicken by adding a quarter of water over a stove in a cooking pot. Use heat and let it boil. Add one tea cubit salt and place in the pot the chicken breasts—cover and boil for 22 minutes in medium heat. Remove from the pot the chicken. Let it cool down. Let it cool down! Shred manually and set aside.

2. Prepare the macaroni using the instructions for the package. Boil in pot three-quarters of water. Add one tea cubicle salt. Give the macaroni into the pot. Stir. Cover the saucepan and keep boiling the macaroni for 9 minutes in medium heat or until al-dente. Take care that the macaroni sticks to every other every 3 minutes. Drain the water. Drain the water. Set aside the macaroni.

3. Put Macaroni in a big bowl of mixing. Add chicken shredded. Toss.

4. Add the choice of lady Mayonnaise and powder of garlic. Toss softly until thoroughly integrated.

NUTRITION: Calories 746 Fat 36g Carbohydrates 75g Protein 25g

288. Ginataang Talong with Malunggay and Tofu

Preparation Time: 5 minutes
Cooking Time: 30 minutes
Servings: 4
INGREDIENTS:

- Prep Time5 minutes
- Cook Time30 minutes
- Ingredients
- Two pieces of eggplants sliced
- 40 grams Knorr Ginataang Gulay Recipe Mix
- 8 ounces extra-firm tofu air fried for 10 minutes
- One cup of Malunggay leaves
- Two cups of water
- One-piece onion chopped
- Four cloves garlic chopped
- Three tbsp cooking oil
- Ground black pepper to taste
- Salt to taste

DIRECTIONS:
1. Sprinkle garlic and onion until soft later.
2. Prepare coconut milk with Knorr Ginataang Gulay Recipe Mix. Mix until the mixture is well mixed.
3. In the pan, pour cocoa milk. Cover and let boil. Cover.
4. Add aubergine. Cover the pot for 8 minutes and cook.
5. Add tofu fried air. Remove and cook for 3 minutes.
6. Fill with Malunggay leaves. Remove and cook for 1 minute.
7. Season with black pepper and salt when necessary. Season.
NUTRITION: Calories 294 Fat 17g Carbohydrates 25g Protein 13g

289. Bicol Express Recipe

Preparation Time: 5minutes
Cooking Time: 55 minutes
Servings: 6
INGREDIENTS:

- 2 lbs. pork belly sliced into strips

- Two cups of coconut milk
- Two cups of coconut cream
- 1/2 cup of shrimp paste bagoong Alamang
- Four cloves garlic crushed
- Six pieces Thai chili pepper chopped
- One thumb ginger minced
- One-piece onion chopped
- One-pieces Serrano pepper sliced
- One cup of water optional

DIRECTIONS:
1. Mix ginger, garlic, onion, Thai chili, pork, and coconut milk in a pot. Turn the heat on and cover the pan.
2. Remove the cover. Remove the cover. Stir. Add half the bagoong and pour One cup of the cocoon and One cup of water into the mixture. Remove and heat to low. Cook till a fourth of the sauce (around 50 minutes).
3. Add the remaining cocoon cream and saucepan (as needed). Add the peppers of Serrano, too. Keep simmering until the sauce thickens (about) at low heat.
4. Serve with warm rice and transfer to a serving platter.
NUTRITION: Calories 1240 Fat 124g Carbohydrates 10g Protein 27g

290. Chicken Gravy

Preparation Time: 3 minutes
Cooking Time: 12 minutes
Servings: 4
INGREDIENTS:

- Three tbsp butter
- Four tbsp all-purpose flour
- One-piece Knorr Chicken Cube
- 1/Two teaspoon onion powder
- 1/Four teaspoon garlic powder
- 1/8 teaspoon ground black pepper
- 1 3/4 cup of water

DIRECTIONS:
1. Melt the gravel in a cup of butter.
2. Add meal for all purposes. Cook for eight minutes in medium heat to form a brown roux.
3. Add Chicken Cube to Knorr. Remove until melted.
4. Put the water into the bowl. Mix until thoroughly mixed. Add the powder of onion, garlic, and ground black pepper. Stir. Cook 1 minute. Cook 1 minute.

NUTRITION: Calories 71 Fat 6g Carbohydrates 4g Protein 1g

291. Crispy Pork Belly Chips

Preparation Time: 1 minute
Cooking Time: 20 minutes
Servings: 6-8
INGREDIENTS:

- 1 ½ lb. pork belly
- Three tbsp Knorr Liquid Seasoning
- 6 cups of water
- Three pieces dried bay leaves
- One teaspoon whole peppercorn

DIRECTIONS:
1. Cover and allow the saucepan to boil. Adjust heat between medium and low. For 60 minutes, continue to cook.
2. Remove the saucepan of pork. Let it cool down.
3. Slice in small pieces. Slice. Note: I usually freeze pork one and ½ an hour before the pig is sliced.
4. Mix pork sliced with liquid seasoning of Knorr. Mix thoroughly. Mix well.
5. Set meat on an air fryer. Put the fryer in the air at 350F and fry the air for 20 minutes or until it is crispy. Note: Make sure the pork slices turn through the middle of the cooking phase. It ensures that both sides are properly cooked.

NUTRITION: Calories 3577 Fat 36g Carbohydrates 8g Protein 70g

292. Chop Suey

Preparation Time: 10 minutes
Cooking Time: 30 minutes
Servings: 5
INGREDIENTS:

- Seven pieces of shrimp cleaned and deveined
- 3 ounces pork sliced
- 3 ounces boneless chicken breast sliced
- 1 ½ cup of cauliflower florets
- One-piece carrot sliced crosswise into thin pieces
- 15 pieces snow peas
- Eight pieces of baby corn
- One-piece red bell pepper cut into squares
- One-piece green bell pepper sliced into squares
- 1 ½ cups of cabbage chopped
- 12 pieces quail eggs boiled
- One-piece yellow onion sliced
- Four cloves garlic crushed
- ¼ cup of soy sauce
- 1 ½ tbsp oyster sauce
- ¾ cup of water
- One tbsp cornstarch diluted in ½ cup of water
- ¼ teaspoon ground black pepper
- Three tbsp cooking oil

DIRECTIONS:
1. In a wok or pan, heat oil.
2. Fry the shrimp on every side for 1 minute. Remove from wok. Remove from wok. Set aside. Set aside.
3. Add garlic and sprinkle until the onion is tender.
4. Add pork and chicken. Remove to light brown.
5. Add soy sauce and sauce to the oyster. Stir.
6. For water. For water. Let boil. Let boil. Cover and simmer for 15 minutes in medium heat.
7. Add cauliflower, carrots, snow peppers, bell peppers, and maize. Stir.
8. Add chicken. Toss. Cover and cook for five to seven minutes.
9. Put the pan-fried shrimp in the pot and add black ground pepper.
10. Add cooked quail eggs and diluted

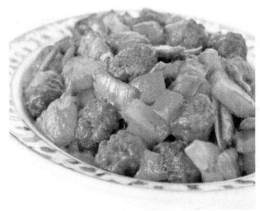

cornstarch to water.

NUTRITION: Calories 214 Fat 13g Carbohydrates 20g Protein 4g

293. Air Fried Fish Sinigang sa Miso

Preparation Time: 10 minutes
Cooking Time: 40 minutes
Servings: 6
INGREDIENTS:

- Two pieces tilapia cleaned
- 40 grams Knorr Sinigang sa Sampaloc Recipe mix
- ¼ cup of miso
- One bunch of mustard leaves
- Eight pieces okra
- One-piece yellow onion wedged
- 6 ounces daikon radish sliced
- Two pieces tomato wedged
- Four pieces long green chili
- 6 to 8 cups of water
- 1/Two teaspoon ground black pepper
- 1 ½ teaspoon cooking oil
- One teaspoon salt
- Fish sauce to taste

DIRECTIONS:

1. Rub salt everywhere, then rub the cooking oil.
2. To cook the fish, use an air fryer. Fry every side for 10 minutes in 350F. Remove and cool. Remove.
3. Put water in a pot. 3. Let it boil. Let it boil.
4. Add onion, tomatoes, radish daikon, and miso. Let the water boil again.
5. Put in the pot the fish. Cook 2 minutes after the water boils again.
6. Add Knorr Sinigang Mix Recipe. Remove.
7. Put into the saucepan the okra and long green peppers. Cover and simmer for 5 minutes in medium heat.
8. Add mustard leaves, then season with black pepper and fish sauce. Cover for three minutes and simmer for three minutes.
9. Transfer to a bowl of pork. Serve.

NUTRITION: Calories 68 Fat 3g Carbohydrates 9g Protein 3g

294. Sweet and Sour Chicken Meatballs

Preparation Time: 10minutes
Cooking Time: 25minutes

Servings: 4
INGREDIENTS:

- One lb. ground chicken
- 1/2 cup of breadcrumbs
- One-piece Knorr Chicken Cube
- One-piece egg
- 1/Four teaspoon salt
- 1/Four teaspoon ground black pepper
- ¼ cup of cooking oil
- One ¾ cup of water
- Four tbsp banana ketchup
- Five tbsp white sugar
- Four tbsp white vinegar
- ¼ cup of bell pepper Julienne
- Two tbsp onion sliced
- Three tbsp carrot Julienne
- One 1/Two tbsp cornstarch diluted in Two tbsp water
- A few drops of Knorr Liquid Seasoning

DIRECTIONS:

1. Make the chicken balls in a large blender with the ground chicken. Grate the chicken cube Knorr piece and add salt and pepper. Crack the egg onto the basin and mix until all contents are mixed. Add breadcrumbs gradually while mixing.
2. Scoop 2 mixture teaspoons. Roll into a figure in a ball shape. Set aside. Set aside. Do this until the whole chicken mixture is finished.
3. Heat pan oil. 3. Fry chicken meatballs every few seconds on medium heat to make them fry evenly. Remove the chicken balls from the saucepan as soon as the outer part becomes brown. Set aside. Set aside.
4. Make the sour sauce. 4. Sprinkle onion with remaining oil until layers are separated. Add carrot and bell pepper. Cook 1 minute. Cook for 1 minute.
5. Pour in water, then add sugar, vinegar, and ketchup banana. 5. Let boil. Remove all ingredients until thoroughly integrated. Remove to obtain desired uniformity.
6. Return the chicken to the pot. Remove to sauce coat.
7. Transfer to the plate of service. Serve. Share and enjoy yourself!

NUTRITION: Calories 445 Fat 25g Carbohydrates31 g Protein 24g

295. Burger Steak

Preparation Time: 10 minutes

Cooking Time: 20 minutes
Servings: 3
INGREDIENTS:

- One lb. ground beef
- One teaspoon onion powder
- One-piece Knorr Beef Cube
- 1/2 cup of breadcrumbs
- 1/Two teaspoon garlic powder
- One-piece egg beaten
- 1/Four teaspoon ground black pepper
- ¼ cup of cooking oil
- Two tbsp parsley chopped
- 5 ounces button mushroom thinly sliced
- Three tbsp butter
- Four tbsp all-purpose flour
- One-piece Knorr Beef Cube
- 1/Four teaspoon Knorr liquid seasoning
- 1/Two teaspoon onion powder
- 1/Four teaspoon garlic powder
- 1 3/4 cup of water

DIRECTIONS:

1. Mix beef pats with ground beef, onion powder, garlic powder, ground black pepper, and egg. 1. Grate 1 Knorr beef cube piece. Mix it all.
2. Make the patties by scooping on the meat mixture in roughly ¼ cup. Mold it into figures formed by balls and flatten.
3. Heat Two tbsp of pan cooking oil. Freeze medium heat on one side of the patties until it is browned. Turn it over and perform the same thing on the other side. Remove from the pot. Remove. Set it aside. Set it away.
4. Make gravy in a saucepan with melted butter.
5. Add all-functional meals—Cook over medium heat and whisk in a brown roux for 8 minutes.
6. Add Knorr Cube Beef. Remove until melted.
7. Put water in the bowl. Stir until thoroughly mixed. Note: you will notice the mixture becoming thicker in time slowly.
8. Add powder onion, garlic, ground black pepper, and liquid seasoning of Knorr. 8. Cook 30 seconds. Cook 30 seconds.
9. Add mushrooms in slices. Cook 1 minute. Cook for 1 minute. Set aside. Set aside.
10. Set beef patties over a cup of steamed rice and then pour beef gravy throughout.

11. Chopped parsley top, 11. Serve warm. Serve
NUTRITION: Calories 400 Fat 32g Carbohydrates 12g Protein 17g

296. Pineapple Chicken Afritada

Preparation Time: 10 minutes
Cooking Time: 50 minutes
Servings: 6
INGREDIENTS:

- 2 lbs. chicken cut into serving pieces
- One-piece Knorr chicken cube
- 8 ounces tomato sauce
- 8 ounces pineapple chunks in a can
- One-piece potato diced
- One-piece carrot sliced
- One-piece red bell pepper cut into squares
- One-piece green bell pepper cut into squares
- One-piece onion chopped
- Four cloves garlic chopped
- Three pieces dried bay leaves
- Three tbsp cooking oil
- One cup of water
- Fish sauce and ground black pepper to taste

DIRECTIONS:

1. Heat pan oil. 1. Add garlic. Add garlic. Continue to cook while mixing until golden brown becomes colored.
2. Fill in onion. Sprinkle until soft.
3. Stir in chicken—Cook for 1 minute on every side or until light brown.
4. In the pan, pour tomato sauce, pineapple juice, and water. Stir. Cover the pan. Cover the pan.
5. Add Knorr Chicken Cube and bay leaves after the liquid starts to boil. Cover the pot and then set the heat to a low level. Keep cooking for 18 minutes.
6. To turn the chicken pieces over, use a tong for the kitchen. Continue to cook for 12 minutes on the opposite side.
7. Pineapples, potatoes, and carrots should be added. Cook 10 minutes. Cook 10 min.
8. Season with ground black pepper and fish sauce.
9. Add pepper bell. 9. Three to five minutes of cooking time.
10. Transfer to a bowl of portions. Serve and please!

NUTRITION: Calories 182 Fat 11g
Carbohydrates 21g Protein 2g

Chapter 17. Complex recipes

297. Mini Key Lime Cheesecake

Preparation Time: 10 minutes
Cooking Time: 25 minutes
Servings: 4
INGREDIENTS:

- ¼ cup lime juice
- 1 small banana
- ¼ teaspoon iodized salt
- 1½ cups macadamia nuts, raw and soaked overnight
- ¼ cup almond milk, unsweetened
- 3¼ tablespoons pure maple syrup, separated
- 1/3 teaspoon pure vanilla extract, sugar-free
- 3¼ tablespoon coconut oil, separated

DIRECTIONS:

1. Empty macadamia nuts into a glass dish the night before you prepare the cheesecake.
2. Remove water from the nuts and transfer ½ a cup to a food blender. Pulse for approximately 60 seconds or until they are a slightly chunky consistency.
3. Combine ¾ tablespoons of coconut oil and maple syrup, along with vanilla extract, salt, and banana. Pulse until the mix becomes a sticky consistency.
4. Transfer the mixture evenly between 4 quiche, pie, or ramekin dishes. Press to create a smooth surface consistently through the pans, then place in the freezer.
5. In the meantime, transfer the leftover macadamia nuts, coconut oil, and maple syrup in a food blender.
6. Blend almond milk and lime juice by pulsing for approximately 45 seconds or until a smooth consistency.
7. Transfer the pie dishes to the countertop and evenly distribute the filling between each. Use a rubber scraper to flatten the filling and create a smooth top.
8. Place the cheesecakes back into the freezer and wait approximately 1 hour or until firm before serving.
9. When ready to serve, take the cheesecakes out of the freezer 10 minutes before enjoying.

NUTRITION: Protein: 3g Carbohydrates: 21g Fat: 37g Calories: 172

298. Mint Mocha Bites

Preparation Time: 10 minutes
Cooking Time: 20 minutes
Servings: 8

INGREDIENTS:

- 1 tablespoons cocoa, unsweetened and powdered, separated
- 4 tablespoons coconut oil, melted
- 1 teaspoon instant coffee*
- 1/3 Cup Stevia sweetener, granulated and separated
- 2 teaspoon hot water
- 1/3 Cup almond flour**
- ¼ tsp. pure mint extract, sugar-free

DIRECTIONS:

1. Empty water into a mug and nuke in the microwave for 30 seconds.
2. Dissolve instant coffee in the hot water.
3. Using a food blender, pulse 4 tablespoons of the Stevia, 1 teaspoon of cocoa powder, 4 tablespoons of coconut oil, and ¼ teaspoon of mint extract until thoroughly combined.
4. Integrate coffee and almond flour until batter thickens.
5. Freeze for approximately 10 minutes.
6. Meanwhile, in a separate glass dish, blend the leftover 4 teaspoons of Stevia and 2 teaspoons of cocoa powder until incorporated.
7. Remove the dish from the freezer and roll into four individual balls.
8. Rotate each ball to coat it completely with the cocoa/Stevia coating and serve immediately.
9. For any leftovers, transfer to the refrigerator in a sealed tub and they will keep fresh for about 5 days.
10. If you choose, you can also use decaffeinated coffee.

NUTRITION: Protein: 1g Carbohydrates: 24g Fat: 7g Calories: 78

299. Dark Chocolate Gelato

Preparation Time: 10 minutes
Cooking Time: 10 minutes
Servings: 16
INGREDIENTS:

- 2 ¼ cups of coconut milk

- ¾ cup lactose-free heavy cream
- 2 tablespoons arrowroot starch
- ½ cup of cocoa powder
- 4 Oz. dark chocolate
- ¾ cup of sugar

DIRECTIONS:

1. In a saucepan, place half of the coconut milk, cream, arrowroot starch, cocoa powder, and dark chocolate. Add in the sugar.

2. Turn on the stove & bring the mixture to a simmer until it thickens. Turn off the heat and add the remaining milk. Mix until well combined.

3. Pour into an ice cream maker. Turn the ice cream maker for 3 hours until the mixture turns into a gelato.

4. If you do not have an ice cream maker, you can place the mixture in a lidded container. Place in the fridge for 8 hrs. But make sure that you mix the mixture every hour to create the creamy gelato texture.

NUTRITION: Calories 145, Total Fat 11.4g, Saturated Fat 9.1g, Total Carbs 11g, Net Carbs 7.5g, Protein 2.5g, Sugar: 3.4g, Fiber: 3.5g, Sodium: 20mg, Potassium: 299mg

300. Bread Pudding with Blueberries

Preparation Time: 10 minutes
Cooking Time: 40 minutes
Servings: 2
INGREDIENTS:

- 1 extra-large egg
- 2/3 cup unsweetened almond milk
- 1 tablespoon maple syrup
- ¼ teaspoon vanilla extract
- 4 slices of gluten-free bread
- ½ cup blueberries
- A dash of ground cinnamon

DIRECTIONS:

1. Preheat the oven to 3750F.

2. In a bowl, almond milk, whisk the eggs, and maple syrup until well combined. Add in the vanilla extract.

3. Cut the crusts from the bread & slice the bread into tiny cubes. Place the bread cubes in a greased baking dish and pour the egg mixture. Top with blueberries and sprinkle with a dash of cinnamon.

4. Bake for 40 minutes or until the egg mixture is set and the top has browned and puffed up.

NUTRITION: Calories 268, Total Fat 6.5g, Saturated Fat 2.6g, Total Carbs 44.9g, Net Carbs 42.8g, Protein 7.8g, Sugar: 25.6g, Fiber: 2.1g, Sodium: 238mg, Potassium: 215mg

301. Chocolate English Custard Recipes

Preparation Time: 10 minutes
Cooking Time: 10 minutes
Servings: 2
INGREDIENTS:

- 1 ½ tablespoon tapioca starch
- 1 egg
- 1 tablespoon pure maple syrup
- ¾ cup almond milk
- 1 tablespoon water
- 1 ½ tablespoon cocoa powder

DIRECTIONS:

1. Add all ingredients in a saucepan and whisk until all lumps are removed.

2. Place the saucepan on the stove and then bring to a boil over low heat while stirring constantly.

3. Turn off the heat once the mixture thickens.

4. Pour into ramekins and refrigerate for 3 hours before serving.

NUTRITION: Calories 170, Total Fat 6.5g, Saturated Fat 2.1g, Total Carbs 24.6g, Net Carbs 21.4g, Protein 5.8g, Sugar: 16.2g, Fiber: 3.2g, Sodium: 340mg, Potassium: 892mg

302. Homemade Chocolate Lollipops

Preparation Time: 15 minutes
Cooking Time: 25 minutes
Servings: 12
INGREDIENTS:

- Lollipop Sticks
- 1 Package bittersweet chocolate chips
- 1 Package white chocolate chips
- 1 Package milk chocolate chips
Assorted Toppings
- Nuts walnuts,
- Dried fruit wild blueberries, tart cherries, chopped apricots, craisins, raisins

- Mini marshmallows
- Candy canes crushed
- Health bars chopped
- Candied ginger chopped
- Seeds sunflower, pumpkin

DIRECTIONS:

1. Prepare all you garnish first. At that point, place chocolate contributes a microwave-safe bowl and microwave on high for 30 seconds. Mix chips at that point microwave again for an additional 30 seconds and blend once more. Rehash this procedure until chocolate is smooth and softened. Do this for each kind of chocolate, and afterward, you are prepared to gather the candies.

2. Gather up liquefied chocolate on an enormous teaspoon and cautiously hold the spoon vertically over the material paper giving the chocolate a chance to drop on to the paper around. Smooth edges as vital with your spoon. Next, place top of a candy stick on liquefied chocolate around 1/3 of the path from the base. Press tenderly into chocolate to verify, at that point improve with garnishes to your deepest longing!

3. Spot preparing sheets in refrigerator to cool. Following 5-10 minutes you will most likely appreciate.

NUTRITION: Calories: 149 Carbs: 17g Protein: 1g Fat: 8g

303. Granola Bars

Preparation Time: 15 minutes
Cooking Time: 15 minutes
Servings: 12
INGREDIENTS:

- 1 cup rice flake
- 1 cup millet flakes
- ½ cup dried cranberries
- ½ cup pumpkin seeds
- ¼ cup sunflower seeds
- ½ cup peanut butter
- 2 teaspoons malt syrup
- 1 teaspoon cinnamon powder
- Coconut oil for greasing

DIRECTIONS:

1. Preheat the oven to 3550F and grease a small baking tray.

2. In a bowl, mix together the rice flakes, millet, cranberries, pumpkin seeds, and peanut butter.

3. In a blender, mix together the peanut butter, and malt syrup. Add in the cinnamon powder.

4. Pour into the granola mixture & mix well.

5. Press into the baking tray and bake for 15 minutes.

6. Allow hardening before cutting into bars.

NUTRITION: Calories 180, Total Fat 8.6g, Saturated Fat 1.4g, Total Carbs 23.4g, Net Carbs 19g, Protein 6.1g, Sugar: 4.4g, Fiber: 4.4g, Sodium: 175mg, Potassium: 270mg

304. Baked Peanut Butter Protein Bars

Preparation Time: 20 minutes
Cooking Time: 0 minutes
Servings: 12
INGREDIENTS:

- 1 cup natural creamy peanut butter
- ¾ cup maple syrup
- 1 teaspoon vanilla bean paste
- 1 ½ cups gluten-free rolled oats
- 1 cup of protein powder

DIRECTIONS:

1. Line a baking pan with parchment paper.

2. In a microwave-safe bowl, heat the peanut butter and maple syrup for 30 seconds. Stir then add in the vanilla bean paste then heat again for 30 seconds.

3. Stir in oats and protein powder.

4. Spread into the prepared pan and press using the back of the spoon.

5. Refrigerate for an hour and cut into 12 bars.

NUTRITION: Calories 271, Total Fat 14.9g, Saturated Fat 2.5g, Total Carbs 27.6g, Net Carbs 23.4g, Protein 14g, Sugar: 13.7g, Fiber: 4.2g, Sodium: 128mg, Potassium: 442mg

305. Lime Cake

Preparation Time: 20 minutes
Cooking Time: 45 minutes
Servings: 8
INGREDIENTS:

- 2 ½ cups gluten-free flour
- 1 tablespoon baking powder
- 1 teaspoon xanthan gum
- 4 large eggs
- 1 cup canola oil
- 1 cup of coconut milk
- 1 teaspoon vanilla extract

- 1 teaspoon lime extract
- 2 cups of sugar
- ½ teaspoon salt
- 1 tablespoon lime zest
- 3 tablespoons freshly squeezed lime juice

DIRECTIONS:

1. Preheat the oven to 3500F and grease a cake pan with shortening or oil.
2. In a large bowl, baking powder, mix the flour, and xanthan gum. Sift through a sieve to aerate the dry ingredients.
3. In another bowl, mix together the eggs, canola oil, coconut milk, vanilla extract, lime extract, sugar, salt, lime zest, and lime juice. Beat until the sugar dissolves, and the liquid turns smooth.
4. Fold in the dry ingredients gradually and mix until the lumps are removed.
5. Pour the batter into the prepared pan. Tap the bottom of the pan to remove too much air within the batter.
6. Place in the oven and bake for 45 minutes.

NUTRITION: Calories 422, Total Fat 30.7g, Saturated Fat 3.4g, Total Carbs 35.2g, Net Carbs 34.9g, Protein 3.1g, Sugar: 26.5g, Fiber: 0.3g, Sodium: 221mg, Potassium: 114mg

306. Chocolate Pavlova with Pomegranate, Raspberries & Kiwi

Preparation Time: 20 minutes
Cooking Time: 2 hours
Servings: 8
INGREDIENTS:

Meringue:
- 4 Ounces (115 g) bittersweet chocolate, finely chopped, preferably at least 60 to 70% cacao
- 4 Large egg whites
- ¼ teaspoon cream of tartar
- 1 Cup (198 g) sugar, preferably superfine
- 2 teaspoons cornstarch
- ½ teaspoon apple cider vinegar
- ½ teaspoon vanilla extract

Topping:
- 1 Cup (240 ml) heavy cream, chilled
- 2 Teaspoons confectioners' sugar
- 3 Tablespoons pomegranate seeds
- 12 Raspberries, very firm and fresh
- 2 Green kiwi, peeled and sliced crosswise into thin rounds

DIRECTIONS:

For the Meringue:

1. Preheat broiler to 250°F/121°C. Line a preparing sheet field with material paper and follow a 9-inch (23 cm) hover on the paper; turn paper over.
2. Dissolve the chocolate until easy and allow to chill to scarcely heat; installed a safe spot.
3. In a great, oil-free bowl whip egg whites with inflatable whip connection of stand blender or utilize an electric powered mixer on low speed till foamy. Include cream of tartar and hold beating, going tempo to high, till delicate pinnacles shape. Include sugar slowly and beat till meringue is hardened and reflexive so that you can take a few minutes. Beat in cornstarch, vinegar, and vanilla.
4. Sprinkle the chocolate over the meringue and in all respects tenderly make more than one folds to deliver chocolate streaks in the course of the meringue. You can OVER blend in all respects effectively. Decide in want of much less.
5. Scoop the meringue onto fabric inside the circle and make use of the returned of a giant spoon to assist shape a spherical plate in the drawn circle, being aware so as not to exhaust the marbling. Make a moderate sorrow inside the focal factor of the circle. You will hear the whipped cream and natural product inside the middle and a downturn within the meringue will assist hold the fixings.
6. A spot in stove and heat for 1 hour 15 minutes, at that point, test the meringue circle. It ought to be sparkling, dry and simply tinged with the faintest degree of shading. Keep heating for 15 minutes more if essential. Mood killer stove and enable the plate to chill inside the broiler. Once cooled, the plate is probably put away in a water/air evidence compartment at room temperature for as long as 3 days.
7. For the Toppings:
8. Whip the cream in a clean and calm bowl with the sugar until the shape of a touchy pinnacle. Spot meringue circle on level presentation platter. Heap the whipped cream inside the focal point of the meringue, permitting a fringe of meringue to stay. Spot natural product over whipped cream, to a wonderful quantity, and serve in (chaotic) wedges with spoons to scoop the whole thing up.

NUTRITION: Calories: 314 Carbs: 44g Protein: 3g Fat: 10g

307. Celery Soup

Preparation Time: 8 Minutes
Cooking Time: 10 Minutes
Servings: 4
INGREDIENTS:

- Olive oil (1 tbs)
- Garlic cloves (3, minced)
- Celery (2 lbs., fresh, chopped into
- One-inch pieces.)
- Vegetable stock (6 cups)
- Salt (1 tsp)

DIRECTIONS:
1. Reserve celery tops for later use. Heat up the oil over medium heat in a soup pot.
2. Cook garlic until softened, about 3-5 minutes. Add celery stalks, salt and vegetable stock and bring to a boil.
3. Cover and reduce heat to low and simmer until celery softens. Let the soup cool for a bit then and puree with a hand blender.
4. Add and cook the celery tops on medium heat for 5 minutes.
NUTRITION: 51 calories, 3 g fat, 4 g carbs, 2 g fiber, 2 g protein

308. Carrot & Turkey Soup

Preparation Time: 15 Minutes
Cooking Time: 40 Minutes
Servings: 4
INGREDIENTS:

- Ground turkey (1/2 lb., lean)
- Frozen carrot (1/2 bag)
- Green peas (1/4 cup)
- Chicken broth (1 can (32 oz)
- Tomatoes (2 medium, seeded, and roughly chopped)
- Garlic powder (1 tsp)
- Paprika (1 tsp)
- Oregano (1 tsp)
- Bay leaf (1)

DIRECTIONS:
1. Over medium heat, brown the ground turkey in a soup pot. Add peas, frozen carrot, paprika, tomatoes, garlic powder, bay leaf, oregano, and broth.
2. Bring pot to a boil, reduce heat, cover, and simmer for 30 minutes.
NUTRITION: 436 calories, 12 g fat, 20 g carbs, 6 g fiber, 59 g protein

309. Shrimp & Pasta Salad

Preparation Time: 15 Minutes
Cooking Time: 12 Minutes
Servings: 2
INGREDIENTS:

- White refined pasta (1/2 lb., shells or tubes)
- Shrimp (3/4 lb. Medium, peeled, deveined, and cooked)
- Fresh spinach (2 cups)
- Roma tomatoes (2 medium, seeded and chopped)
- Light ranch salad dressing (1/2 cup)
- Basil (4 tbs, chopped coarsely)
- Parmesan cheese (1/4 cup, grated)

DIRECTIONS:
1. Bring a salted water to boil in a pot. Cook the pasta as the package instructed. Drain the water from the pasta.
2. In a bowl, combine cooked pasta, spinach, salad dressing, tomatoes and shrimp. Refrigerate for 20 minutes.
3. Toss together with basil and cheese. Serve.
NUTRITION: 516 calories, 20 g fat, 55 g carbs, 7 g fiber, 32 g protein

310. Baked Chicken Breasts

Preparation Time: 5 Minutes
Cooking Time: 15 Minutes
Servings: 4
INGREDIENTS:

- 4 boneless, skinless chicken breasts
- 2 tbsp. Extra Virgin Olive Oil
- 1 tsp. kosher salt
- 1/2 tsp. black pepper 1/2 tsp garlic powder
- 1/2 tsp. onion powder
- 1/2 tsp. chili powder

DIRECTIONS:
1. Turn your oven on and allow to preheat up to 450 degrees F. Lightly grease a 9x13-inch baking dish.
2. Pound the chicken breasts until they are an even ¾-inch thick. Lightly coat the chicken with olive oil.
3. Whisk together the salt, pepper, garlic powder, onion powder and chili powder.
4. Season the chicken on both sides with the spice mixture and place in the prepared pan.

5. Set to bake in the preheated oven for about 20 minutes (checking after the 15-minute mark), or until the chicken is cooked through.

6. Rest for 5-10 minutes, covered with foil, then slice and serve.

NUTRITION: 205 calories, 10 g fat, 1 g carbs, 3 g fiber, 27 g protein

311. Dump Pot Chicken & Rice

Preparation Time: 10 Minutes
Cooking Time: 25 Minutes
Servings: 4
INGREDIENTS:

- Chicken white meat (1 lb., strips)
- 2 cups cooked basmati rice
- Water (1/4 cup)
- Soy sauce (1/4 cup, low sodium)
- Lemon juice (1/2 cup))
- Extra-virgin olive oil (3 tbsp.)
- ½ tsp salt
- ¼ tsp ground pepper
- 2 tbsp. Chives, finely chopped

DIRECTIONS:

1. Combine the water, soy sauce and lemon in a small bowl. Mix well.

2. Heat 2 Tbs olive oil and cook the chicken over medium high heat in a skillet until cooked through.

3. Add the soy mixture. Simmer for 15 minutes to reduce the sauce. Add in the remaining ingredients, except chives, and season to taste.

4. Continue to cook for 4-5 minutes, or until the rice is heated through. Garnish with chives and serve.

NUTRITION: 177 calories, 1 g fat, 31 g carbs, 1 g fiber, 11 g protein

312. Italian Inspired Chicken Skillet

Preparation Time: 10 Minutes
Cooking Time: 20 Minutes
Servings: 4
INGREDIENTS:

- Chicken breasts (4 large, boneless skinless cut 1/4-inch thin)
- Dried oregano (1 tbsp., divided)
- Salt (1 tsp)
- Black pepper (1 tsp., divided)
- Olive oil (3 tbsp.)
- Baby Bella mushrooms (8 oz., cleaned, trimmed, and sliced)
- Grape tomatoes (14 oz., halved)
- Garlic (2 tbsp., fresh, chopped)
- Chicken or vegetable stock (1/2 cup)
- Lemon juice (1 tbsp., freshly squeezed)
- Chicken broth (3/4 cup)
- Handful baby spinach (optional)

DIRECTIONS:

1. Season the chicken on both sides with half of the oregano, salt and pepper.

2. Heat 2 Tbs of oil in a heavy skillet and brown the chicken on both sides for 3 minutes.

3. Remove the chicken and set aside. Sauté the mushrooms in the same skillet, add another tablespoon of oil if needed.

4. Add the tomatoes, garlic and remaining oregano, salt and pepper.

5. Cook for another 3 minutes. Deglaze the pan with the chicken or vegetable stock and then stir in the chicken broth and lemon juice.

6. Bring the liquid to a boil and then return the chicken to the pan.

7. Reduce heat to medium and simmer for 8-10 minutes, or until the chicken is fully cooked and the liquid is reduced to desired consistency.

8. Serve with rice or quinoa, if desired.

NUTRITION: 278 calories, 11 g fat, 12 g carbs, 8 g fiber, 34 g protein

313. Turkey Burgers with Cucumber Salad

Preparation Time: 15 Minutes
Cooking Time: 15 Minutes
Servings: 4
INGREDIENTS:

- Turkey burgers:
- Turkey (1 lb., lean ground)
- Egg (1 large, beaten)
- Oatmeal (½ cup)
- Onions (1/3 cup, grated)
- Parsley (1/3 cup, finely chopped)
- Garlic (1 clove, minced)
- Sea salt (½ tsp)
- Black pepper (½ tsp)
- Olive oil (1 tbsp., extra-virgin)
- Canola oil (2 tsp.)
- Cucumber salad:

- Cucumber (1, diced small)
- Chives (1/2 cup, chopped)
- Ripe tomato (1 medium, finely diced)
- Freshly squeezed lime or lemon juice (2 tbsp.)
- ¼ tsp kosher or sea salt

DIRECTIONS:

1. Combine the turkey burger ingredients, except oil, and mix well. Form into 4 patties.
2. Lightly grease the grill and grill the patties for 5-6 minutes per side on medium high.
3. Meanwhile, combine the cucumber salad ingredients and chill until serving.

NUTRITION: 314 calories, 0 g fat, 15 g carbs, 3 g fiber, 26 g protein

314. Saltfish Salad

Preparation Time: 30 Minutes
Cooking Time: 0 Minutes
Servings: 4
INGREDIENTS:

- Salted cod (1 lb.)
- Yellow onion (1 large, thinly sliced)
- Tomato (1 large, diced)
- Eggs (3 hard-boiled, quartered)
- Green olives (12, optional)
- Olive oil (1/4 cup)
- Chicken or vegetable stock (1 tbsp.)

DIRECTIONS:

1. Soak the cod in cold water for 15-30 minutes. Drain and place in a large pot. Cover the cod with water and bring to a boil.
2. Change the water and bring to a simmer another 3-4 times, or until the cod is reduced to the appropriate saltiness.
3. Drain and break the cod into pieces. Sauté the onion with olive oil for 5-6 minutes, or until soft.
4. Add all your ingredients to a bowl then mix until it is fully combined. Serve with rice and drizzled with olive oil.

NUTRITION: 613 calories, 28 g fat, 9 g carbs, 4 g fiber, 78 g protein

Chapter 18. Snacks

315. Banana-bread muffins
Preparation time: 15 minutes
Cooking time: 30 minutes
Servings: 12
Ingredients:

- 2 cups oat flour
- 1 teaspoon baking soda
- Pinch sea salt
- 1 tablespoon ground cinnamon
- ½ cup coconut oil
- 3 unripe bananas, mashed
- 2 eggs
- ¾ cup raw sugar
- ¼ cup maple syrup
- ½ teaspoon pure vanilla extract
- ½ cup chopped walnuts or pecans
- ½ cup blueberries

Directions:

1. Preheat the oven to 325°f. Line a muffin tin with paper liners.
2. Combine the oat flour, baking soda, salt, and cinnamon in a medium bowl. Set aside.
3. In a small microwave-safe bowl, melt the coconut oil in the microwave. Pour it into a large mixing bowl and add the mashed bananas, eggs, sugar, maple syrup, and vanilla. Mix well.
4. Add the dry ingredients to the wet ingredients, and stir until well combined. Gently fold in the walnuts and blueberries.
5. Fill each muffin cup three-quarters full. Bake for 25 to 30 minutes, or until a toothpick inserted into the center of a muffin comes out clean.

Nutrition: calories: 213; carbohydrates: 29g; fat: 11g; protein: 2g; fiber: 2g; sodium: 135mg

316. Berry fruit leathers
Preparation time: 5 minutes
Cooking time: 3 hours and 30 minutes
Servings: 6
Ingredients:

- 2 cups strawberries
- 2 cups blueberries
- ½ cup maple syrup
- Juice of 1 lemon

Directions:

1. Preheat the oven to 200°f. Line two baking sheets with parchment paper.
2. Add the strawberries, blueberries, maple syrup, and lemon juice to a blender, and blend until smooth.
3. Divide the mixture between the two small baking sheets and use a rubber spatula to spread it across the sheets in an even layer.
4. Bake for 3 to 3½ hours, or until no longer sticky when you tap it with your finger.
5. Let the berry leather cool for about 30 minutes, then use a pizza cutter or scissors to cut it into 8 strips, each about 1 inch wide and 5 inches long.

Nutrition: calories: 38; carbohydrates: 11g; fat: 0g; protein: 0.5g; fiber: 1g; sodium: 2mg

317. Chocolate-covered banana slices
Preparation time: 10 minutes
Cooking time: 5 minutes
Servings: 2
Ingredients:

- 1 unripe banana, frozen and sliced
- ½ cup high-quality milk- or dark-chocolate chips

Directions:

1. Line a baking sheet with parchment paper and place the banana slices on the sheet in a single layer so that they're not touching each other.
2. In a microwave-safe bowl, melt the chocolate in the microwave at 30-second intervals, making sure to stir it between intervals.
3. Pour the chocolate over the banana slices so they're completely covered.
4. Refrigerate for at least 1 hour so the chocolate hardens completely. Transfer to an airtight container and refrigerate for up to 1 week.

Nutrition: calories: 333; carbohydrates: 46g; fat: 20g; protein: 5g; fiber: 6g; sodium: 1mg

318. Coconut macaroons
Preparation time: 10 minutes
Cooking time: 15 minutes
Servings: 12
Ingredients:

- 6 egg whites
- Pinch sea salt
- ½ cup maple syrup
- 1 tablespoon vanilla extract
- 3 cups unsweetened shredded coconut

Directions:
1. Preheat the oven to 350°f. Line two baking sheets with parchment paper.
2. In a small bowl, add the egg whites and salt. Using an electric mixer on high speed, whisk the eggs until firm peaks form, 5 to 6 minutes.
3. Using a rubber spatula, gently fold in the maple syrup, vanilla, and coconut until well combined.
4. Drop 1 rounded tablespoon of batter at a time on the baking sheet, leaving about 2 inches between each macaroon.
5. Bake for 12 to 15 minutes, or until lightly browned.

Nutrition: calories: 156; carbohydrates: 13g; fat: 10g; protein: 3g; fiber: 2g; sodium: 42mg

319. Banana ice cream

Preparation time: 5 minutes
Cooking time: 0 minutes
Servings: 2
Ingredients:
- 2 frozen bananas
- 2 tablespoons cocoa powder
- 2 tablespoons peanut butter
- 1 teaspoon maple syrup
- ½ teaspoon vanilla extract

Directions:
Put the frozen bananas, cocoa powder, peanut butter, maple syrup, and vanilla in a blender, and blend until smooth. Serve immediately or freeze in an airtight, freezer-safe container.

Nutrition: calories: 111; carbohydrates: 18g; fat: 5g; protein: 3g; fiber: 3g; sodium: 38mg

320. Berry berry sorbet

Preparation time: 30 minutes
Cooking time: 0 minutes
Servings: 2
Ingredients:
- 1 cup halved strawberries
- 1 cup blueberries
- Juice of 1 lemon

- 1/3 cup maple syrup

Directions:
1. In a blender, add the strawberries, blueberries, lemon juice, and maple syrup. Blend until the mixture has a smooth and even texture.
2. Pour the mixture into an ice cream maker and freeze the sorbet according to the manufacturer's instructions. It takes about 25 minutes.
3. Transfer the sorbet into an airtight, freezer-safe container and let freeze for at least 2 hours before serving.

Nutrition: calories: 104; carbohydrates: 26g; fat: 0g; protein: 1g; fiber: 2g; sodium: 5mg

321. Oatmeal semisweet chocolate-chip cookies

Preparation time: 15 minutes
Cooking time: 11 minutes
Servings: 12
Ingredients:
- 2½ cups oat flour
- 1 teaspoon baking soda
- Pinch sea salt, plus extra for garnish
- ½ cup coconut oil
- 2/3 cup dark brown sugar
- 1 egg
- 1 teaspoon vanilla extract
- ½ cup semisweet chocolate chips

Directions:
1. Preheat the oven to 350°f. Line two baking sheets with parchment paper.
2. In a medium bowl, combine the oat flour, baking soda, and salt. Set aside.
3. In a microwave-safe bowl, melt the coconut oil in a microwave, then pour it into a large mixing bowl.
4. To this large bowl, add the sugar, egg, and vanilla. Mix until well combined.
5. Add the dry ingredients to the wet ingredients and mix well.
6. Fold in the chocolate chips until just combined.
7. Put tablespoon-size scoops of batter on the baking sheets, leaving about 2 inches between each cookie. Bake for about 11 minutes, or until golden brown.

8. As soon as the cookies come out of the oven, sprinkle them with a little salt. Let the cookies cool on the pan for about 2 minutes, then transfer them to a wire rack to cool completely.

Nutrition: calories: 93; carbohydrates: 9g; fat: 6g; protein: 1g; fiber: 1g; sodium: 67mg

322. Coconut-lemon bars

Preparation time: 40 minutes
Cooking time: 32 minutes
Servings: 12
Ingredients:
For the crust

- Nonstick cooking spray
- 1½ cups old-fashioned oats
- ½ cup unsweetened shredded coconut
- ¼ cup raw sugar
- Pinch sea salt
- ¼ cup coconut oil

For the filling

- 2 eggs
- ½ cup raw sugar
- 5 tablespoons freshly squeezed lemon juice
- 1 tablespoon freshly grated lemon zest
- 1 teaspoon vanilla extract
- 2 tablespoons cornstarch
- For the topping
- 1/3 cup raw sugar
- ¼ cup freshly squeezed lemon juice
- ¼ cup water
- 2 tablespoons cornstarch
- ¼ cup unsweetened shredded coconut

Directions:
To make the crust

1. Preheat the oven to 350°f. Spray an 8-by-8-inch baking pan with the cooking spray.
2. In a food processor, add the oats, coconut, and sugar. Process until they're combined and ground to a fine texture.
3. In a microwave-safe bowl, melt the coconut oil in a microwave. Add the melted coconut oil to the food processor, and pulse until it's combined with the oat mixture.
4. Transfer the mixture to the baking pan and press it down with the back of a spoon until it covers the bottom of the pan in an even layer.

5. Bake for about 14 minutes, or until golden brown. Set aside to cool for at least 20 minutes.

To make the filling

1. While the crust is cooling, add the eggs to the bowl of a stand mixer. Beat on medium-high speed for 2 to 3 minutes, until the eggs are light and foamy.
2. Add the sugar, lemon juice, lemon zest, and vanilla, and continue mixing until completely combined, about 1 minute.
3. Put ¼ cup of the egg mixture in a small bowl and whisk in the cornstarch. Add that back into the bowl of the stand mixer, and whisk well until fully incorporated.
4. Pour the filling into the cooled crust. Bake for 18 minutes, or until the top is no longer wet.
5. To make the topping
6. While the filling and crust are baking, in a small saucepan over medium heat, add the sugar, lemon juice, water, and cornstarch. Heat, stirring frequently, until the mixture thickens, 2 to 3 minutes. Stir in the coconut and remove the pan from the heat.
7. Pour the topping over the baked lemon bars and gently spread it across into an even layer.
8. Chill the pan in the refrigerator for at least 1 hour before slicing.

Nutrition: calories: 251; carbohydrates: 30g; fat: 14g; protein: 3g; fiber: 3g; sodium: 37mg

323. Flourless chocolate cake with berry sauce

Preparation time: 20 minutes
Cooking time: 30 minutes
Servings: 10

Ingredients:
For the cake

- ½ cup (or 1 stick) unsalted butter, chopped, plus additional for greasing the pan
- 6 ounces dark chocolate, chopped
- 2 egg whites
- ¾ cup white sugar
- 3 eggs
- ½ cup high-quality unsweetened cocoa powder, sifted

For the berry sauce

- 2 cups frozen strawberries
- 2 cups blueberries
- 1/3 cup maple syrup
- 2 tablespoons freshly squeezed lemon juice

Directions:

To make the cake

1. Preheat the oven to 350°f.
2. Grease the bottom and sides of a 9-inch round cake pan with butter, line the bottom of the pan with parchment paper, and grease the top of the paper with more butter.
3. Using a double boiler or a heatproof bowl nestled over a pot of boiling water, melt the chocolate and ½ cup of butter until smooth, stirring frequently. Remove from the heat and set aside.
4. Using an electric mixer, beat the egg whites on medium-high speed until soft peaks form, about 3 minutes. With the mixer running, slowly add the sugar, and mix until just combined.
5. In a large bowl, whisk together the eggs and cocoa powder until just combined.
6. Pour the melted-chocolate mixture into the egg mixture and stir to combine. Then gently fold the egg whites into the batter until just combined, making sure not to overmix. Pour the batter into the cake pan.
7. Bake for about 30 minutes, rotating the pan once after 15 minutes. The cake is ready once it's set in the center and begins to pull away from the sides of the pan. Let the cake cool completely before removing it from the pan.
8. To make the berry sauce
9. Put the strawberries, blueberries, maple syrup, and lemon juice in a medium saucepan over medium-high heat. Use the back of a spoon to break down the berries into smaller pieces as they heat. Constantly stir the sauce until it begins to bubble and thicken, 2 to 3 minutes.
10. Remove the saucepan from the heat and let the sauce cool before serving.

Nutrition: calories: 296; carbohydrates: 42g; fat: 16g; protein: 5g; fiber: 4g; sodium: 37mg

324. **Baked parsnip chips**

Preparation time: 5 minutes
Cooking time: 30 minutes

Servings: 4
Ingredients:

- 3 parsnips
- ½ teaspoon extra-virgin olive oil
- Pinch sea salt
- Freshly ground black pepper

Directions:

1. Preheat the oven to 375°f. Line a baking sheet with parchment paper.
2. Using the slicing blade of a food processor (or a mandolin slicer), thinly slice the parsnips, leaving the skin on.
3. In a large bowl, gently mix the sliced parsnips, olive oil, salt, and pepper, until the slices are coated on both sides.
4. Place the parsnip slices in an even layer on the baking sheet, making sure they don't overlap. Bake for 15 minutes, flip over the chips, and bake for 15 minutes more, or until golden brown and crispy.

Nutrition: calories: 79; carbohydrates: 18g; fat: 1g; protein: 1g; fiber: 5g; sodium: 49mg

325. **Lemon ricotta cake (crepe cake recipe)**

Preparation Time: 20 minutes
Cooking Time: 25 minutes
Total time: 45 minutes
Servings: 16
Ingredients:

For the ricotta cream filling

- 1/4 cups heavy cream
- 1/2 cup granulated sugar
- Teaspoon vanilla extract
- 32 oz ricotta cheese

For the strawberry sauce

- 3 cups fresh strawberries, hulled and divided
- 1/3 cup strawberry jam
- Pinch salt
- Chopped pistachios, optional garnish

For the crepe batter

- Tablespoons melted butter
- 2/3 cups whole milk
- 1/4 cups water
- 2 1/2 cups all-purpose flour
- 3 tablespoons granulated sugar
- 1/2 teaspoons salt

- 5 large eggs
- Zest of 1 lemon + 1 tablespoon juice

Directions:

For the ricotta cream filling

1. In a mixing bowl, combine the ricotta cheese. Fill a vita-mix blender container halfway with heavy cream, sugar, and vanilla extract. Cover and push the "start" button at level 1. Increase the speed of the machine to level 10 by turning it on. For gentle peaks, blend for 10-15 seconds. Don't over mix, or you'll end up with churned butter!

2. Scoop the whipped cream from the blender jar and mix it gently into the ricotta cheese with a spatula. (if you put the ricotta in the blender, it will crumble.) Place in the refrigerator until ready to use.

For the strawberry sauce

1. Rinse the blender jar well. To the jar, add 2 cups cut strawberries, strawberry jam, and a sprinkle of salt: blend and cover. Begin with level 1 and gradually increase the speed until the strawberries are dissolved. Refrigerate the strawberry sauce in a small jar until ready to serve.

For the crepe batter

1. Rinse the blender jar well. Combine the flour, sugar, salt, eggs, milk, water, melted butter, 1 lemon zest, and 1 tablespoon lemon juice in a mixing bowl. Cover and mix for 5 seconds on level 1. Then, gradually raise the speed to level 10, until the mixture is foamy. If there are visible flour clumps, scrape the jar's edges. Then, cover and mix for another 5-10 seconds.

2. Over medium heat, heat a 9- to 10-inch flat nonstick crepe pan. Once the pan is heated, spoon batter into the center of the crepe pan with a 1/4-cup scoop. Lift and swirl the pan quickly to form a thin 9-inch circle of batter. Return the pan to the stovetop. If you're having problems forming uniform circles, use a spatula to transfer the batter to the pan's sparse spots swiftly.

3. Cook for 30-40 seconds on each side, turning with a broad flat spatula. The first side should have a light golden hue with golden speckles, and the second side should be lighter. Turn the heat up to medium-high if your crepes are taking longer than 90 seconds total per crepe.

4. Repeat with the remaining crepes on a baking sheet (or plate) coated with parchment paper. The crepes will be brittle at first, but they will soften in a matter of minutes. You should have 20-24

crepes. It is ok to stack them on the sheet. They will not cling together if they are thoroughly cooked.

5. Before proceeding, allow the crepes to cool fully. To expedite the chilling process, place the baking sheet in the refrigerator.

To assemble

1. Begin building the cake after the crepes have completely cooled. One crepe should be placed on a cake stand. Spread 1/4 cup ricotta filling in a thin circle over the crepe, leaving a 1/2-inch ring around the edges without cream. Repeat with the remaining crepes. Spread ricotta cream and stack crepes until all of the ricotta filling and/or crepes are used. To level out the layers, use a flat plate or baking sheet to push down on the top of the cake. Cover loosely with plastic wrap and keep refrigerated until ready to serve.

To serve

1. Slice the remaining 1 cup fresh strawberries and put them on top of the cake. Pour some of the strawberry sauce over the strawberries, allowing it to drip down the edges. The leftover sauce should be reserved for pouring over individual slices of cake. If desired, decorate the top of the cake with chopped pistachios.

2. When it's time to cut the cake, use a serrated knife and make nice, even slices with a gently sawing motion. Serve with more strawberry sauce.

Nutrition facts: calories: 349 | carbohydrates: 53 g | protein: 48 g | fat: 2 g | cholesterol: 284 mg

326. Sweet fried plantains

Preparation Time: 5 minutes
Cooking Time: 5 minutes
Total time: 10 minutes
Servings: 6

Ingredients:

- 3 very ripe plantains yellow with lots of blacks
- 6 tablespoons butter
- Clove garlic smashed
- Salt

Directions:

1. Remove the plantain tips. Peel the plantains and cut them into 12 inch thick ovals at an angle.

2. Preheat a big sauté pan or cast iron skillet to medium heat. Then, on the side, place a "holding plate" lined with paper towels.

3. Melt the butter in the pan. Once the butter has melted, add the crushed garlic clove and plantain pieces in a single layer to the pan. (depending on the size of your pan, you may need to do this in two batches.) Fry the plantains until golden brown, about 2-3 minutes per side.

4. When the plantains are golden and crisp, transfer them to a holding plate with a slotted spoon. Season generously with salt. If necessary, repeat with the remaining plantains.

5. Remove the garlic clove. Warm it up with your favorite mexican or caribbean dishes!

Notes: be careful to use plenty of ripe plantains... They should be dark or have big black dots if they are fully ripe. When eaten immediately after being fried, fried plantains offer the finest texture and flavor. However, when they've cooled, you may store leftover plantains in an airtight jar in the fridge for up to 3 days. Reheat in the oven, toaster, or on the stovetop. I do not advocate freezing fried sweet plantains.

Nutrition facts: calories: 210 | carbohydrates: 29 g | protein: 17 g | fat: 22 g | cholesterol: 187 mg

327. French chocolate silk pie recipe

Preparation Time: 30 minutes
Cooking Time: 15 minutes
Total time: 45 minutes
Servings: 10

Ingredients:
• Unbaked pie crust, store-bought or homemade
• 6 oz bittersweet chocolate + extra for shavings
• 1/2 cups of heavy cream
• One cup of unsalted butter softened (2 sticks)
• One cup of granulated sugar, divided
• ½ teaspoons of vanilla extract
• 1/2 teaspoon of salt
• Large pasteurized eggs
Directions:

1. Preheat the oven to 375 degrees fahrenheit. Fill a large 9-inch pie pan halfway with pie dough. The edges should be crimped. Then, cover the pie shell with parchment paper and fill it with dry beans or ceramic pie weights. Cook for 15-20 minutes, or until the edges are golden brown. Allow the pie crust to cool fully after removing the parchment containing the weights.

2. Meanwhile, in a double boiler, melt 6 oz of chocolate. When the chocolate has melted, remove it from the heat and let it cool to room temperature.

3. In the bowl of an electric mixer, combine the heavy cream and 1/4 cup sugar. Whip the cream on high with a whip attachment until it forms firm peaks. Place the whipped cream in a separate dish and set aside until ready to use.

4. Using the same mixer bowl and a paddle attachment, beat the butter and 3/4 cup sugar on high for at least 3 minutes, or until light and fluffy. Turn the heat to low and gradually add the cooled chocolate to the butter mixture, vanilla, and salt. Scrape down the mixer bowl and continue to beat until smooth.

5. Increase the speed of the mixer to high. Add 1 egg at a time, allowing the mixer to beat the egg for at least 3 minutes before adding the next egg. This results in a super-smooth texture. After 12 minutes on high, switch off the mixer. Using a spatula, gently fold in 1/3 of the whipped cream. Fold until the mixture is smooth.

6. Fill the cooled pie shell with the chocolate mixture. Serve with the remaining whipped cream on top. Then, using a vegetable peeler, shave chocolate over the top. Refrigerate for at least 3 hours, or until the chocolate filling has firmed up.

Nutrition facts: calories: 549 | carbohydrates: 30 g | protein: 54 g | fat: 28 g | cholesterol: 197 mg

328. Peanut butter oatmeal chocolate chip cookies (monster cookie recipe)

Preparation Time: 15 minutes
Cooking Time: 15 minutes
Total time: 30 minutes
Servings: 55

Ingredients:
• 5 ½ cups rolled oats (gluten free)
• 5 large eggs

- ¼ cup water
- 2 tablespoons of vanilla extract
- One cup of unsalted butter, softened (2 sticks)
- ¾ cups peanut butter, crunchy or creamy
- ½ cups granulated sugar
- ½ cups light brown sugar, packed
- ½ cup all-purpose flour (or gf baking flour)
- 4 tablespoon baking powder
- 1 teaspoon salt
- 12 ounce semi-sweet chocolate chips
- 12 ounce m&ms

Directions:

1. Preheat the oven to 350 degrees fahrenheit. Set aside several baking sheets lined with parchment paper.
2. Measure out the oats in a large mixing basin. Then, crack the eggs into the oats and stir in the water and vanilla extract. Allow the liquid to soak the oats before stirring to coat.
3. Add the butter to the bowl of an electric stand mixer. To soften, beat for 1 minute. After that, stir in the peanut butter and both sugars. To break down the sugar crystals, beat on high for 3-5 minutes.
4. Scrape down the sides of the bowl with a spatula and beat again to incorporate.
5. Mix in the flour, baking powder, and salt with the mixer on low. Begin adding the oat mixture once everything has been thoroughly combined.
6. Scrape the bowl one more, then mix in the chocolate chips on low.
7. Finally, using a spatula, fold the m&ms into the dough.
8. To distribute the cookie dough onto the prepared baking sheets, use a big 3 tablespoon cookie scoop. Place the cookies 2 inches apart on a baking sheet.
9. Bake for 15-17 minutes each batch, or until the edges are just starting to turn golden brown. Cool for 3 minutes on the baking sheets before transferring.

Nutrition facts: calories: 230 | carbohydrates: 26 g | protein: 4 g | fat: 7 g | cholesterol: 18 mg

100-day meal plan

Days	Breakfast	Lunch	Dinner
1	APPLE ORANGE JUICE	BANANA OAT SHAKE	CHICKEN BONE BROTH
2	PINEAPPLE MINT JUICE	BANANA-APPLE SMOOTHIE	HOMEMADE BEEF STOCK
3	CELERY APPLE JUICE	BERRYLICIOUS SMOOTHIE	THREE-INGREDIENT SUGAR-FREE GELATIN
4	HOMEMADE BANANA APPLE JUICE	BUTTERMILK HERB RANCH DRESSING	CRANBERRY-KOMBUCHA JELL-O
5	SWEET DETOX JUICE	CITRUS RELISH	STRAWBERRY GUMMIES
6	PINEAPPLE GINGER JUICE	CHICKPEA PANCAKES RECIPE	FRUITY JELL-O STARS
7	CARROT ORANGE JUICE	RED WINE SANGRIA RECIPE	SUGAR-FREE CINNAMON JELLY
8	STRAWBERRY APPLE JUICE	SALTY DOG COCKTAIL RECIPE	HOMEY CLEAR CHICKEN BROTH
9	AUTUMN ENERGIZER JUICE	SIMPLE SYRUP	OXTAIL BONE BROTH
10	ASIAN INSPIRED WONTON BROTH	ROSE SANGRIA RECIPE	CHICKEN BONE BROTH WITH GINGER AND LEMON
11	MUSHROOM, CAULIFLOWER AND CABBAGE BROTH	CHAMPAGNE HOLIDAY PUNCH RECIPE	VEGETABLE STOCK
12	INDIAN INSPIRED VEGETABLE STOCK	WHITE SANGRIA	CHICKEN VEGETABLE SOUP
13	BEEF BONE BROTH	RASPBERRY MOJITOS WITH BASIL	CARROT GINGER SOUP
14	GINGER, MUSHROOM AND CAULIFLOWER BROTH	MARGARITA RECIPE	TURKEY SWEET POTATO HASH
15	FISH BROTH	GRAPEFRUIT BASIL SORBET	CHICKEN TENDERS WITH HONEY MUSTARD SAUCE

16	CLEAR PUMPKIN BROTH	BRULEED GRAPEFRUIT (PAMPLEMOUSSE BRÛLÉ)	CHICKEN BREASTS WITH CABBAGE AND MUSHROOMS
17	HEALTHIER APPLE JUICE	FROZEN BEERITAS RECIPE	DUCK WITH BOK CHOY
18	CITRUS APPLE JUICE	SPICY PINEAPPLE HABANERO MARGARITAS	BEEF WITH MUSHROOM AND BROCCOLI
19	RICHLY FRUITY JUICE	CRANBERRY POMEGRANATE MARGARITA WITH SPICED RIM	BEEF WITH ZUCCHINI NOODLES
20	DELISH GRAPE JUICE	PEACH MILKSHAKE (COPYCAT CHIK-FIL-A PEACH SHAKE RECIPE!)	SPICED GROUND BEEF
21	LEMONY GRAPE JUICE	JUGO VERDE (GREEN JUICE)	GROUND BEEF WITH VEGGIES
22	HOLIDAY SPECIAL JUICE	PERFECT MANHATTAN RECIPE	GROUND BEEF WITH GREENS AND TOMATOES
23	VITAMIN C RICH JUICE	FROZEN COCONUT MOJITO	DINNER
24	INCREDIBLE FRESH JUICE	MULLED LEMONADE RECIPE	ITALIAN STYLED STUFFED ZUCCHINI BOATS
25	FAVORITE SUMMER LEMONADE	CUCUMBER ROSE APEROL SPRITZ	CHICKEN CUTLETS
26	ULTIMATE FRUITY PUNCH	PINK GRAPEFRUIT MARGARITA	SLOW COOKER SALSA TURKEY
27	THIRST QUENCHER SPORTS DRINK	STRAWBERRY MARGARITA RECIPE	SRIRACHA LIME CHICKEN AND APPLE SALAD
28	REFRESHING SPORTS DRINK	LARGE-BATCH GOOMBAY SMASH CARIBBEAN COCKTAILS	PAN-SEARED SCALLOPS WITH LEMON-GINGER VINAIGRETTE

29	PERFECT SUNNY DAY TEA	HEALTHY VEGAN BROWNIES	ROASTED SALMON AND ASPARAGUS
30	NUTRITIOUS GREEN TEA	GREEN CHICKEN SOUP	ORANGE AND MAPLE-GLAZED SALMON
31	SIMPLE BLACK TEA	GREEN RISOTTO RECIPE	COD WITH GINGER AND BLACK BEANS
32	LEMONY BLACK TEA	PULAO RICE PRAWNS	HALIBUT CURRY
33	METABOLISM BOOSTER COFFEE	BARBECUE BEEF STIR-FRY	CHICKEN CACCIATORE
34	BREAKFAST LOW FIBER	CHICKEN SAFFRON RICE PILAF	CHICKEN AND BELL PEPPER SAUTE
35	SPINACH FRITTATA	STIR-FRY GROUND CHICKEN AND GREEN BEANS	CHICKEN SALAD SANDWICHES
36	BANANA AND PEAR PITA POCKETS	STEWED LAMB	ROSEMARY CHICKEN
37	RIPE PLANTAIN BRAN MUFFINS	PULLED CHICKEN SALAD	GINGERED TURKEY MEATBALLS
38	EASY BREAKFAST BRAN MUFFINS	LEMONGRASS BEEF	TURKEY AND KALE SAUTE
39	APPLE OATMEAL	BEETROOT CARROT SALAD	TURKEY WITH BELL PEPPERS AND ROSEMARY
40	BREAKFAST BURRITO WRAP	CRUNCHY MAPLE SWEET POTATOES	MUSTARD AND ROSEMARY PORK TENDERLOIN
41	ZUCCHINI OMELET	VEGGIE BOWL	THIN-CUT PORK CHOPS WITH MUSTARDY KALE
42	COCONUT CHIA SEED PUDDING	POMEGRANATE SALAD	BEEF TENDERLOIN WITH SAVORY BLUEBERRY SAUCE
43	SPICED OATMEAL	DIJON ORANGE SUMMER SALAD	GROUND BEEF CHILI WITH TOMATOES

44	BREAKFAST CEREAL	PULAO RICE PRAWNS	FISH TACO SALAD WITH STRAWBERRY AVOCADO SALSA
45	SWEET POTATO HASH WITH SAUSAGE AND SPINACH	WHITE RADISH CRUNCH SALAD	BEEF AND BELL PEPPER STIR-FRY
46	CAJUN OMELET	APPLE AND MUSHROOM SOUP	VEGGIE PIZZA WITH CAULIFLOWER-YAM CRUST
47	STRAWBERRY CASHEW CHIA PUDDING	SPRING WATERCRESS SOUP	TOASTED PECAN QUINOA BURGERS
48	PEANUT BUTTER BANANA OATMEAL	OYSTER SAUCE TOFU	SIZZLING SALMON AND QUINOA
49	OVERNIGHT PEACH OATMEAL	POTATO AND ROSEMARY RISOTTO	BEAN AND HAM SOUP
50	MEDITERRANEAN SALMON AND POTATO SALAD	CHEESY BAKED TORTILLAS	GRILLED PEAR CHEDDAR POCKETS
51	CELERY SOUP	SMOKY RICE	CHICKEN AND APPLE KALE WRAPS
52	PEA TUNA SALAD	ZUCCHINI LASAGNA	CAULIFLOWER RICE PILAF
53	VEGETABLE SOUP	GREEK CHICKEN SKEWERS	FRESH HERB AND LEMON BULGUR PILAF
54	CARROT AND TURKEY SOUP	ROAST BEEF	CORN CHOWDER
55	CREAMY PUMPKIN SOUP	BANANA CAKE	STRAWBERRY AND RHUBARB SOUP
56	CHICKEN PEA SOUP	GRILLED FISH STEAKS	CHICKEN SANDWICHES
57	COCONUT PANCAKES	APPLE PUDDING	TEX-MEX BEAN TOSTADAS
58	BREAKFAST HIGH FIBER	LAMB CHOPS	FISH TACOS
59	MANGO GINGER SMOOTHIE	EGGPLANT CROQUETTES	CUCUMBER ALMOND GAZPACHO

60	CHERRY SPINACH SMOOTHIE	CUCUMBER EGG SALAD	PEA AND SPINACH CARBONARA
61	BANANA CACAO SMOOTHIE	PORK MEDALLIONS WITH ASPARAGUS AND COCONUT CURRY	SAUTÉED BROCCOLI WITH PEANUT SAUCE
62	SPINACH AND EGG SCRAMBLE WITH RASPBERRIES	HIGH-FIBER DUMPLINGS	EDAMAME LETTUCE WRAPS BURGERS
63	BLACKBERRY SMOOTHIE	PIZZA MADE WITH BAMBOO FIBERS	PIZZA STUFFED SPAGHETTI SQUASH
64	VEGGIE FRITTATA	VEGETARIAN HAMBURGERS	SPINACH AND ARTICHOKE DIP PASTA
65	CHOCOLATE BANANA PROTEIN SMOOTHIE	PORK STEAKS WITH AVOCADO	GRILLED EGGPLANT
66	COCOA ALMOND FRENCH TOAST	CHICKEN WITH ASPARAGUS SALAD	STUFFED POTATOES WITH SALSA AND BEANS
67	MUESLI WITH RASPBERRIES	HOT PEPPER AND LAMB SALMON	MUSHROOM QUINOA VEGGIE BURGERS
68	MOCHA OVERNIGHT OATS	PORK ROLLS À LA RATATOUILLE	TURKEY MEATBALLS
69	BAKED BANANA-NUT OATMEAL CUPS	PEPPER FILLET WITH LEEK	SWEET POTATO SOUP
70	PINEAPPLE GREEN SMOOTHIE	LAMB CHOPS WITH BEANS	MINESTRONE SOUP
71	PUMPKIN BREAD	FILLET OF BEEF ON SPRING VEGETABLES	LENTIL SOUP
72	BANANA-BRAN MUFFINS	BOLOGNESE WITH ZUCCHINI NOODLES	GRILLED CORN SALAD
73	BANANA BREAD	CHICKEN WITH CHICKPEAS	KALE SOUP

74	CHOCOLATE-RASPBERRY OATMEAL	HAM WITH CHICORY	PASTA FAGIOLI
75	CHAI CHIA PUDDING	PORK MEDALLIONS WITH ASPARAGUS AND COCONUT CURRY	SWEET POTATO GNOCCHI
76	APPLE CINNAMON OATMEAL	LAMB WITH CARROT AND BRUSSELS SPROUTS SPAGHETTI	BEAN AND HAM SOUP
77	APPLE BUTTER BRAN MUFFINS	CABBAGE WRAP	CHICKEN BONE BROTH
78	PINEAPPLE RASPBERRY PARFAITS	VEAL WITH ASPARAGUS	HOMEMADE BEEF STOCK
79	BERRY CHIA PUDDING	SALMON WITH SESAME SEEDS AND MUSHROOMS	THREE-INGREDIENT SUGAR-FREE GELATIN
80	SPINACH AVOCADO SMOOTHIE	STUFFED TROUT WITH MUSHROOMS	CRANBERRY-KOMBUCHA JELL-O
81	STRAWBERRY PINEAPPLE SMOOTHIE	SALMON WITH BASIL AND AVOCADO	STRAWBERRY GUMMIES
82	PEACH BLUEBERRY PARFAITS	LEEK QUICHE WITH OLIVES	FRUITY JELL-O STARS
83	RASPBERRY YOGURT CEREAL BOWL	FRIED EGG ON ONIONS WITH SAGE	SUGAR-FREE CINNAMON JELLY
84	AVOCADO TOAST	QUINOA MUSHROOM RISOTTO	HOMEY CLEAR CHICKEN BROTH
85	LOADED PITA POCKETS	VEGETARIAN LENTIL STEW	OXTAIL BONE BROTH
86	PEAR PANCAKES	LEMON CHICKEN SOUP WITH BEANS	CHICKEN BONE BROTH WITH GINGER AND LEMON
87	ALMOND PANCAKES	BANANA OAT SHAKE	VEGETABLE STOCK
88	AVOCADO PANCAKES	BANANA-APPLE SMOOTHIE	CHICKEN VEGETABLE SOUP

89	STRAWBERRY PANCAKES	BERRYLICIOUS SMOOTHIE	CARROT GINGER SOUP
90	CARAMBOLA PANCAKES	BUTTERMILK HERB RANCH DRESSING	TURKEY SWEET POTATO HASH
91	GINGER MUFFINS	CITRUS RELISH	CHICKEN TENDERS WITH HONEY MUSTARD SAUCE
92	CARROT MUFFINS	CHICKPEA PANCAKES RECIPE	CHICKEN BREASTS WITH CABBAGE AND MUSHROOMS
93	BLUEBERRY MUFFINS	RED WINE SANGRIA RECIPE	DUCK WITH BOK CHOY
94	COCONUT MUFFINS	SALTY DOG COCKTAIL RECIPE	BEEF WITH MUSHROOM AND BROCCOLI
95	RAISIN MUFFIN	SIMPLE SYRUP	BEEF WITH ZUCCHINI NOODLES
96	PARMESAN OMELETE	ROSE SANGRIA RECIPE	SPICED GROUND BEEF
97	ASPARAGUS OMELET	CHAMPAGNE HOLIDAY PUNCH RECIPE	GROUND BEEF WITH VEGGIES
98	ONION OMELET	WHITE SANGRIA	GROUND BEEF WITH GREENS AND TOMATOES
99	OLIVE OMELETE	RASPBERRY MOJITOS WITH BASIL	CUCUMBER ALMOND GAZPACHO
100	TOMATO OMELET	MARGARITA RECIPE	ITALIAN STYLED STUFFED ZUCCHINI BOATS

Conclusion

Diverticula are small pouches that usually develop from the large intestine after long-standing periods of constipation or straining on the toilet. The pouches can become filled with stool or inflammation and create a blockage in the gut, which can cause severe pain and other symptoms such as nausea, fever, vomiting, constipation, or diarrhea.

There are two types of diverticulitis, an acute or chronic presentation of diverticulitis, with the former being more common. The chronic type is more serious, requiring hospitalization. Diverticular disease can be diagnosed by imaging studies such as sonograms, with the most common finding being a small pouch or sac in the gastrointestinal tract that appears to move periodically.

Acute diverticulitis occurs when the presence of diverticula develops suddenly, with symptoms usually appearing within 6 to 12 hours after straining on the toilet, with most cases occurring in people less than age 50 years. Symptoms are similar to other conditions that involve inflammation and injury of tissue due to trauma or infection, such as appendicitis and peritonitis.

In chronic diverticulitis, the cause is unknown. The condition may be a complication of another condition such as colon cancer, inflammatory bowel diseases, infection of the colon, or medications. It can also be a result of a genetic predisposition. This type usually happens in older people and has a higher mortality rate. Both types may also occur together as part of diverticulosis. In some cases, the pouches will require surgery to remove them. The condition can be treated with medication as well as other methods such as diet changes to improve bowel health and prevent a recurrence.

Diet is an important part of diverticulitis. The aim is to prevent recurrence by avoiding foods that may worsen or cause symptoms such as those with high sugar content such as fruit and processed vegetables, spicy foods, fatty foods, and alcohol; these include red meat and processed meat products. Other food choices for diverticulitis include fish and dairy products.

An important aspect of a healthy lifestyle and immune system is to do regular exercise. It is essential to move the bowels daily and make sure they stay clean and open. Bacteria can live in our intestines for years without causing any symptoms; we only notice them when we get sick or suffer from complications such as diverticulitis. This also means that there is plenty of time to do something about diverticulitis, but you must be healthy in the first place.

To prevent and treat disease, we need to have a thorough understanding of the diseases themselves. We have to know what they are, their causes, and how they work in a state of health. If we understand them in this way, it will be easier to defend our health by preventing disease and by fighting it when it occurs. It is important that we do not let ignorance become a barrier to progress. It is a fact that science cannot answer all our questions about health and disease, but we do know enough to be able to prevent and treat most diseases.

As you have read, there are many causes of diverticulitis. It is hard to get a complete overview of all the factors involved in this very complex disease. When scientists discover more about diverticulitis, this book will be updated. In the meantime, we must recognize that everything in life is connected and related in some way.

Made in the USA
Monee, IL
01 July 2022

98897077R00096